Anorexia and Bulimia Nervosa

Edited by Hubertus Himmerich and Ignacio Jáuregui Lobera

Published in London, United Kingdom

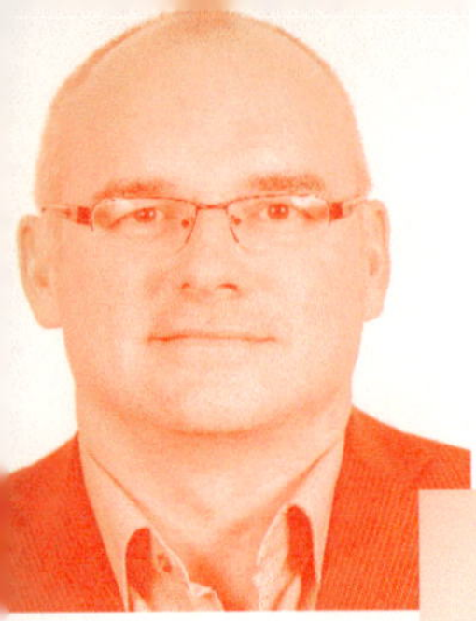
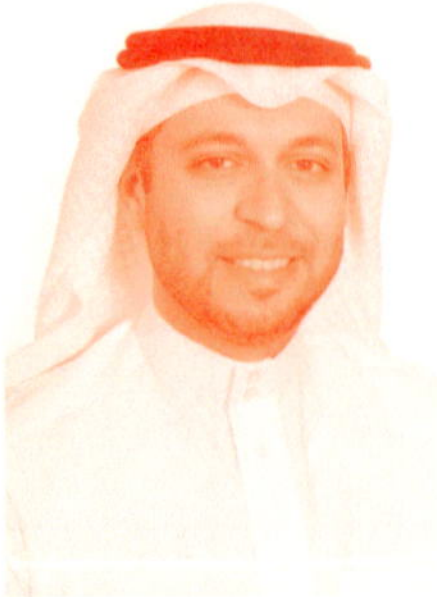
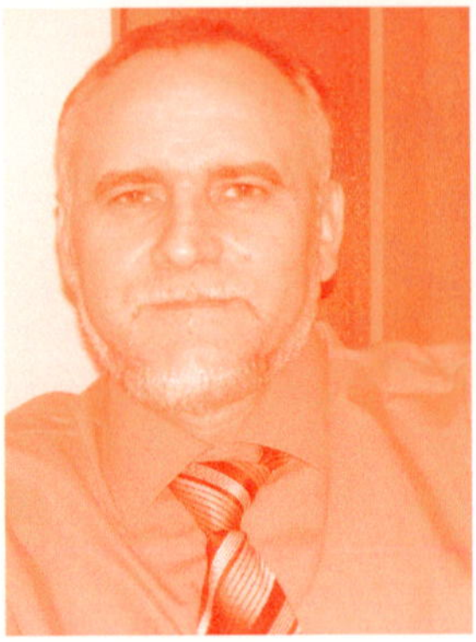
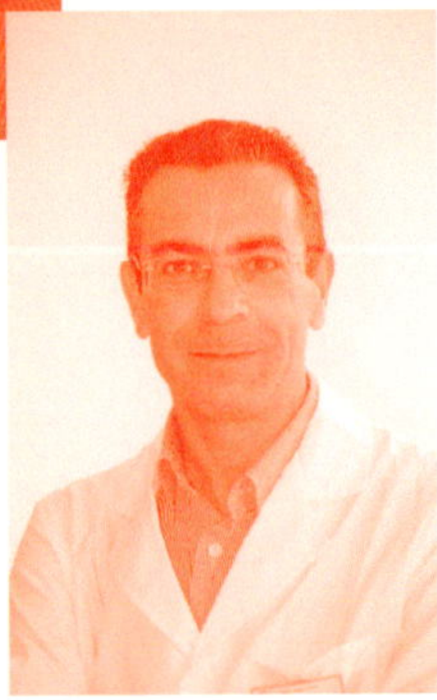
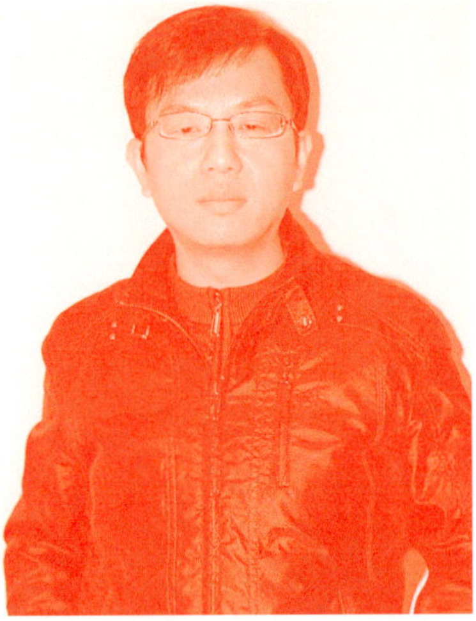
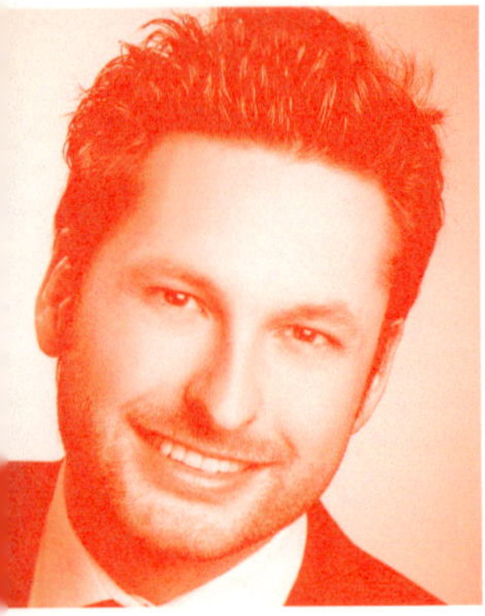
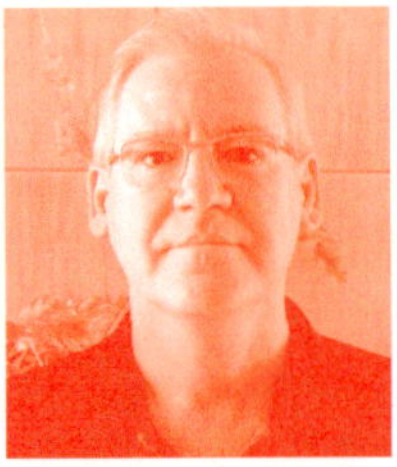

IntechOpen

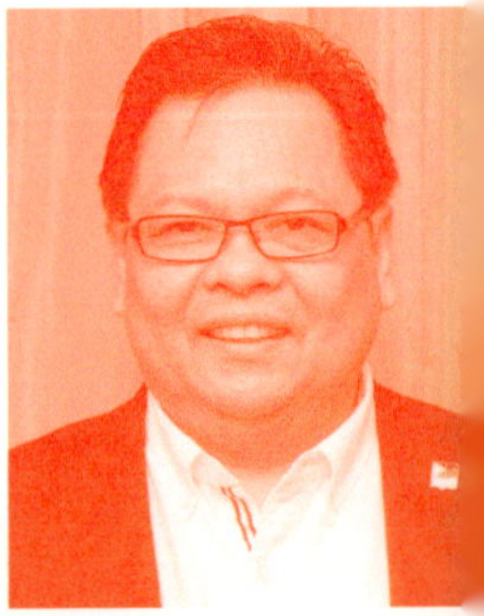
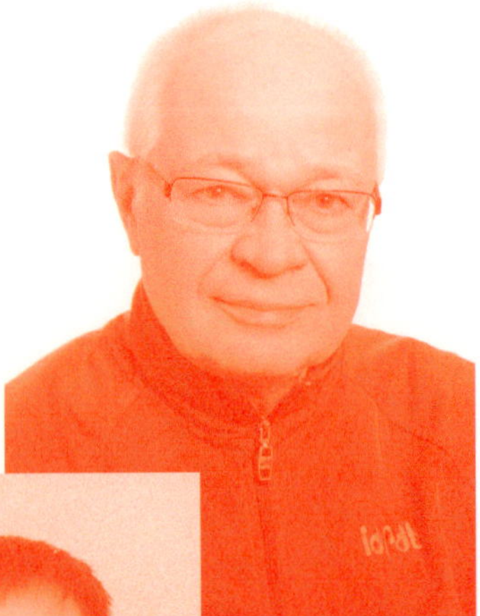
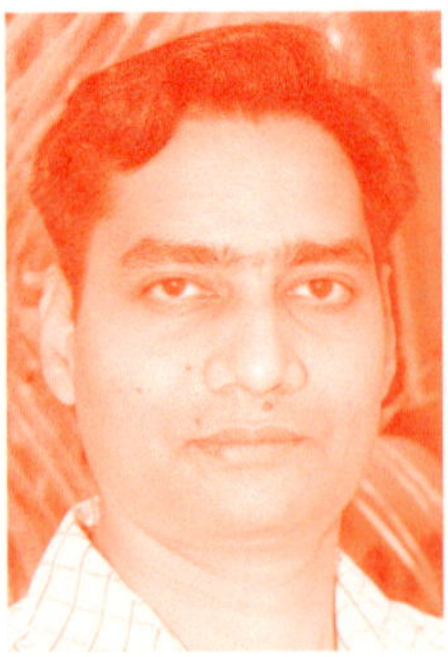
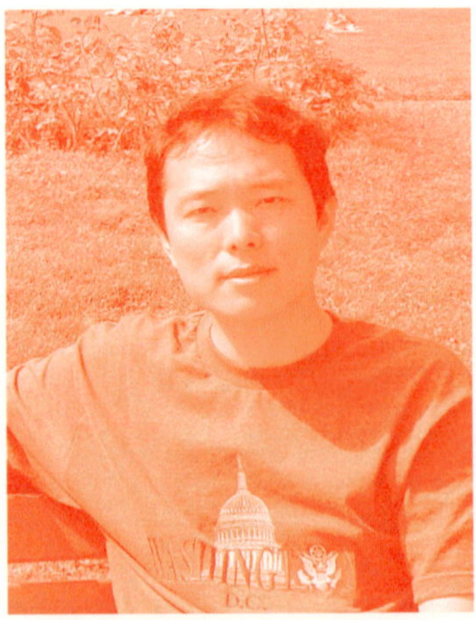
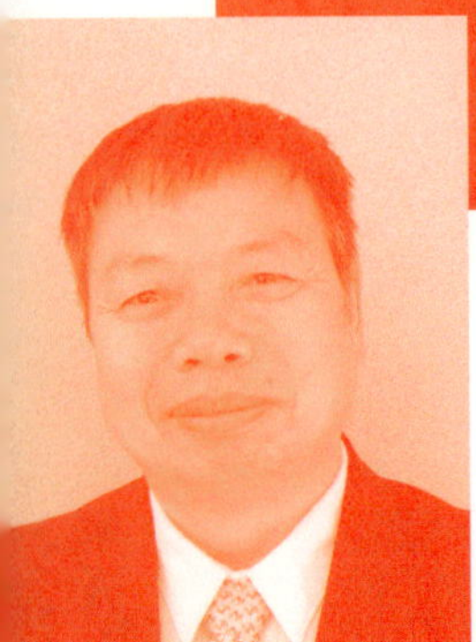
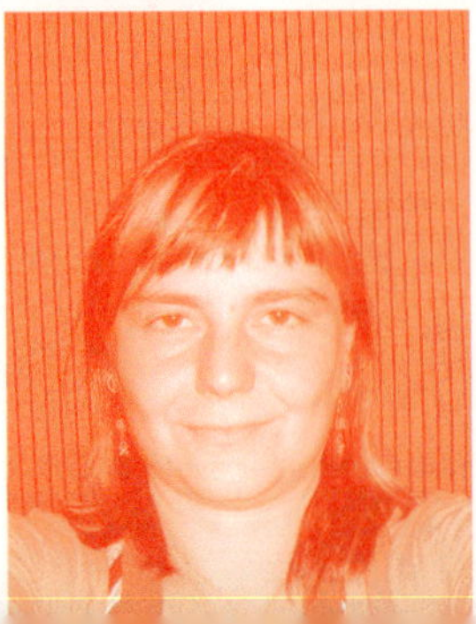

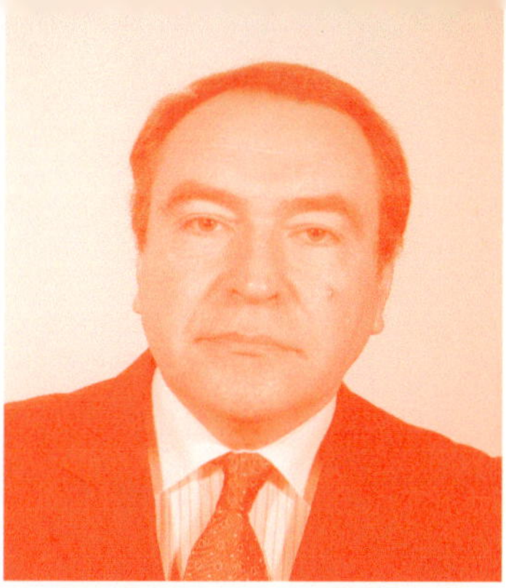

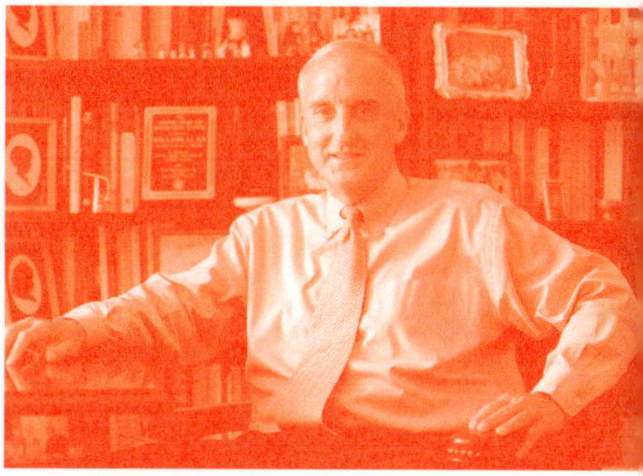

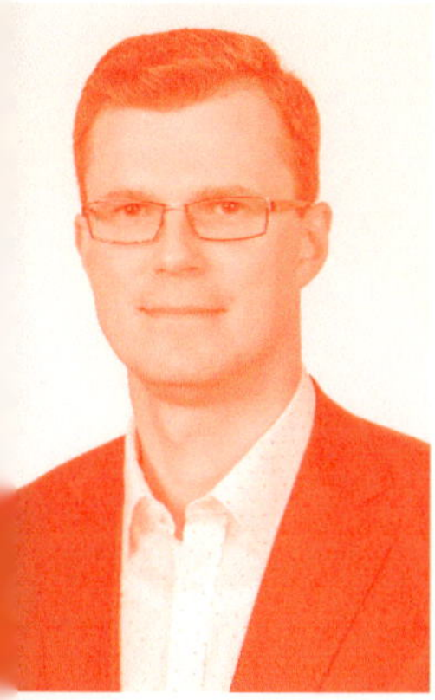

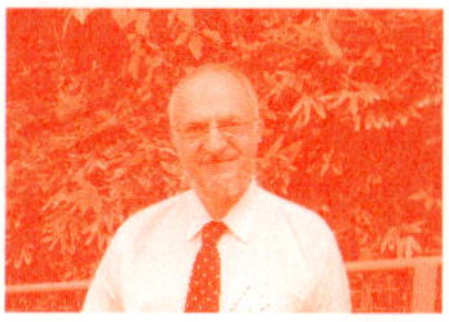

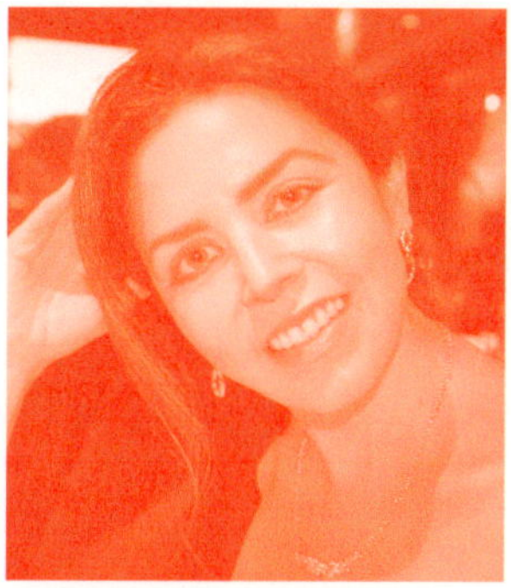

Supporting open minds since 2005

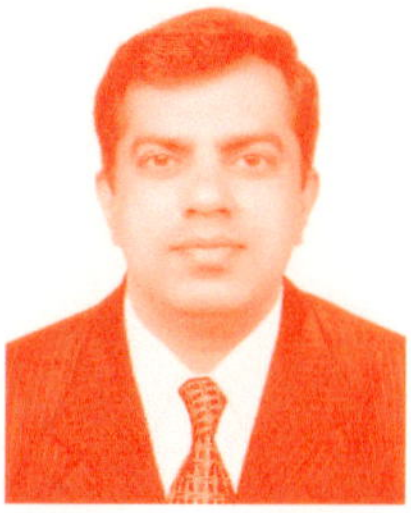

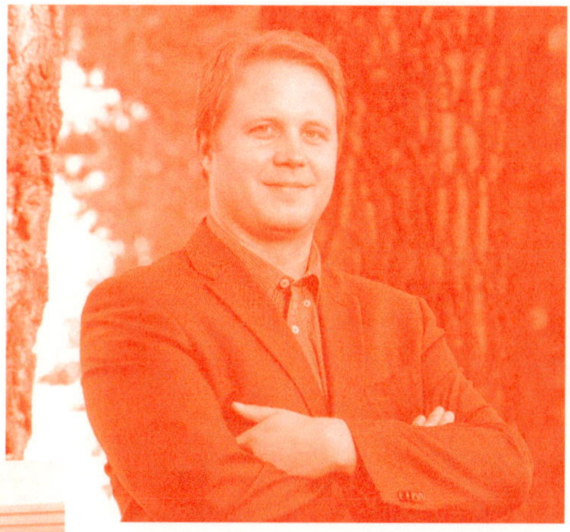

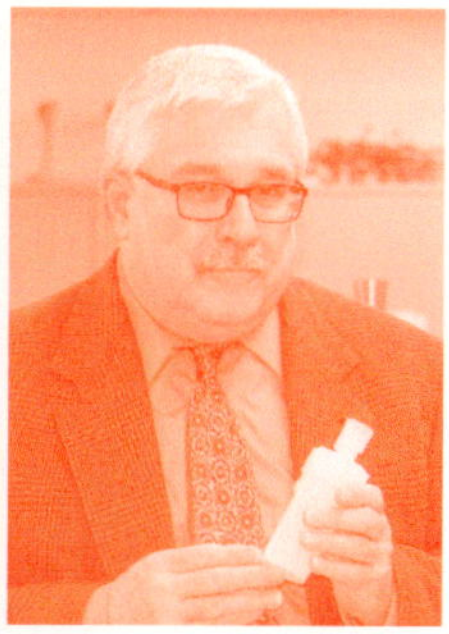

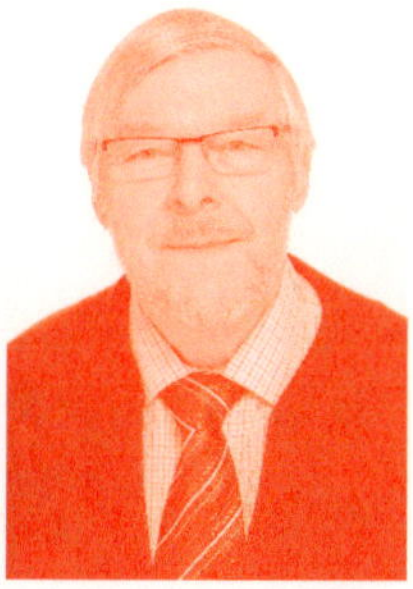

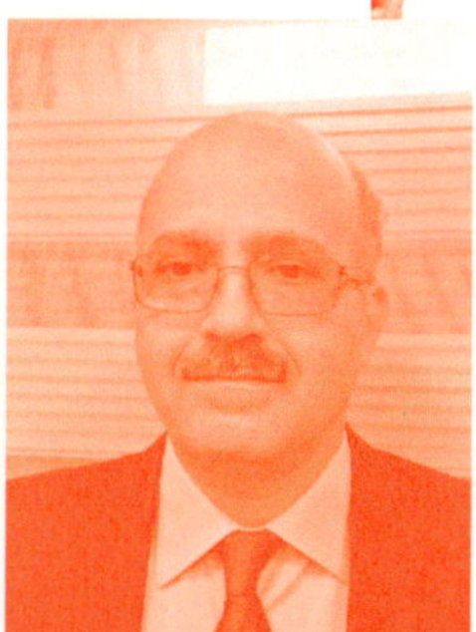

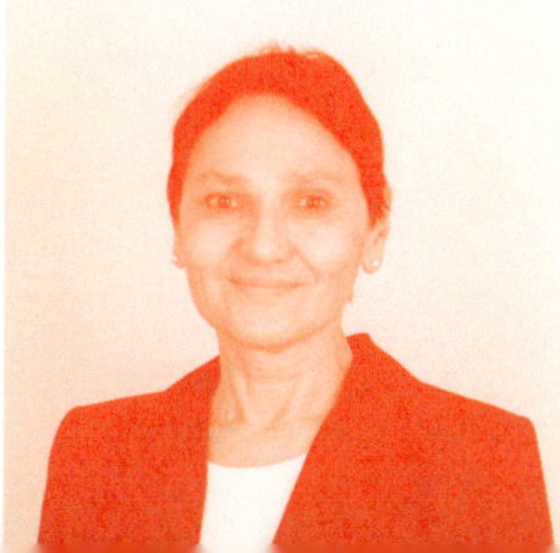

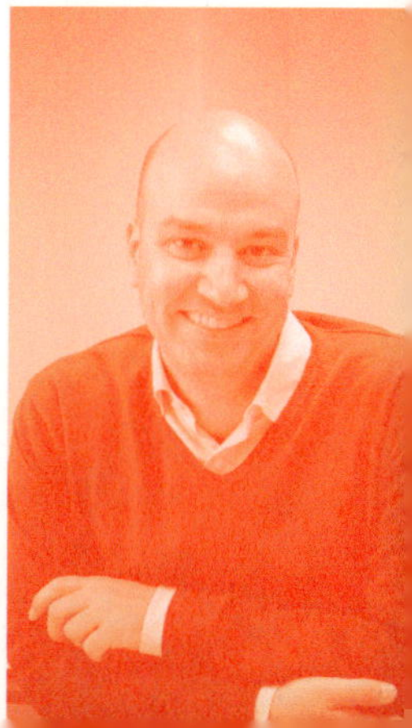

Anorexia and Bulimia Nervosa
http://dx.doi.org/10.5772/intechopen.77704
Edited by Hubertus Himmerich and Ignacio Jáuregui Lobera

Contributors
Samantha Brooks, Helgi Schioth, Marcela Morales-Mulia, Sandra Morales-Mulia, Ashley Higgins, Natalia Solano Pinto, Raquel Fernández-Cézar, Miriam Valles Casas, Anitha Layam, Abigail H. Natenshon, José Vicente Martínez Quiñones, M Martínez Gamarra, Ignacio Jáuregui Lobera, Amabel Dessain, Jessica Bentley, Janet Treasure, Ulrike Schmidt, Hubertus Himmerich, Magnus Sjogren, Stein Frostad, Kenneth Klingenberg_Barfod, Paul Robinson

First published in London, United Kingdom, 2019 by IntechOpen
IntechOpen is the global imprint of INTECHOPEN LIMITED, registered in England and Wales, registration number: 11086078, The Shard, 25th floor, 32 London Bridge Street
London, SE19SG – United Kingdom
Printed in Croatia

British Library Cataloguing-in-Publication Data
A catalogue record for this book is available from the British Library

Additional hard and PDF copies can be obtained from orders@intechopen.com

Anorexia and Bulimia Nervosa
Edited by Hubertus Himmerich and Ignacio Jáuregui Lobera
p. cm.
Print ISBN 978-1-78923-981-2
Online ISBN 978-1-78923-982-9
eBook (PDF) ISBN 978-1-83962-247-2

For EU product safety concerns:
IN TECH d.o.o., Prolaz Marije Krucifikse Kozulić 3, 51000 Rijeka, Croatia, info@intechopen.com or visit our website at intechopen.com.

Meet the editors

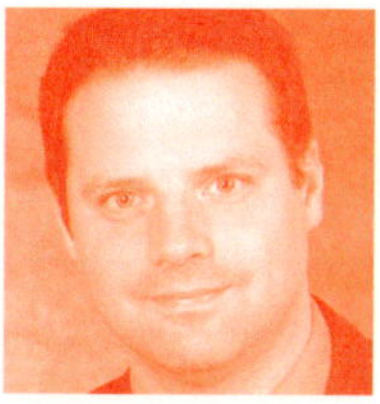

Professor Dr. med. Hubertus Himmerich is a Clinical Senior Lecturer in Eating Disorders at King's College London and a Consultant Psychiatrist on an inpatient ward for patients with eating disorders at the Bethlem Royal Hospital in London, UK. He received his scientific and clinical training at the Max-Planck-Institute of Psychiatry in Munich and the Universities of Mainz and Marburg, Germany. In 2009 he was appointed Professor for Neurobiology of Affective Disorders at the University of Leipzig, Germany. His scientific focuses include appetite regulation, psychoimmunology, and military mental health. He has led and performed national and international scientific projects with researchers from Europe, Australia, and North America, and has published more than 130 articles in peer-reviewed scientific journals as well as a number of books and book chapters.

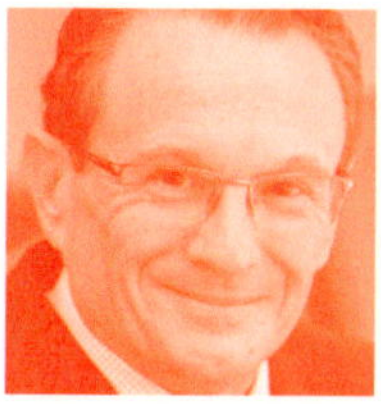

Ignacio Jáuregui-Lobera MD, PsyD, MSc is Director of the Behavioural Science Institute (Seville, Spain) and Associate Professor at Pablo de Olavide University (Seville, Spain). He is the director of the postgraduate course in Eating Disorders and Obesity at the same university. Dr. Jáuregui-Lobera developed his career as a psychiatrist, family practitioner, and psychologist, working in the field of eating disorders and obesity since 1993. He is author of several books and book chapters and more than 100 scientific articles.

Contents

Preface

Although anorexia and bulimia nervosa are two distinct mental illnesses, they are both eating disorders that share common clinical features and symptoms, including the pursuit of weight loss and dissatisfaction with and misperception of body image. They are frequently associated with the same comorbidities, which include affective and anxiety disorders. Therefore, it seems only natural to explore and discuss these closely related diagnoses within the same volume.

This book is divided into four sections. The first section addresses clinically relevant features and symptoms in anorexia and bulimia nervosa. The second section is concerned with the neurobiology of anorexia nervosa and provides novel insights into its pathophysiology and the development of novel medications that target the microbiome for the treatment of eating disorders. The third section focusses on the perspectives of patients and their caregivers, and on family support. The final section highlights and discusses specific aspects related to the clinical management of patients with anorexia and bulimia nervosa.

We are proud to announce that this book has received international contributions from Denmark, India, Mexico, Saudi Arabia, Spain, the United Kingdom, and the United States of America; and we thank all authors for their contributed chapters, which are both informative and offer inspiration.

We would also like to thank IntechOpen and, specifically, Ms. Ivana Barac, Ms. Martina Brkljačić, and Ms. Martina Jošavac for making this book possible.

Hubertus Himmerich
Department of Psychological Medicine,
King's College London,
London, UK

Ignacio Jáuregui-Lobera
Behavioural Science Institute and University of Pablo de Olavide of Seville,
Seville, Spain

Section 1

Features and Symptoms: Impulsivity, Compulsivity, Ambivalence and Body Dissatisfaction

Chapter 1

Impulsivity and Compulsivity in Anorexia Nervosa: Cognitive Systems Underlying Variation in Appetite Restraint from an RDoC Perspective

Samantha Jane Brooks and Helgi Schiöth

Abstract

Contemporary nomenclature for anorexia nervosa (AN) describes the eating disorder as transdiagnostic, with overlapping facets of impulsivity and compulsivity contributing to variations in binge-purge, restrictive eating and maladaptive cognitions. It is important to understand how these facets interact, given that those diagnosed with AN often fluctuate and relapse–as opposed to maintaining a stable diagnosis—between Diagnostic and Statistical Manual version 5 (DSM-5) categories, over the life course. The National Institute of Health's Research Domain Criteria (NIH RDoC) subscribes to the transdiagnostic view of mental disorders and provides progressive guidelines for neuroscience research. As such, using the RDoC guidelines may help to pinpoint how impulsivity and compulsivity contribute to the cognitive mechanisms underlying variations in appetite restraint in eating disorders and common psychiatric comorbidities such as anxiety and obsessive-compulsive disorder. Exploring impulsivity and compulsivity in AN from the perspective of the RDoC cognitive systems domain is aided by measures of genetic, molecular, cellular, neural, physiological, behavioural and cognitive task paradigms. Thus, from the standpoint of the RDoC measures, this chapter will describe some of the ways in which impulsivity and compulsivity contribute to the cognitive systems associated with appetite restraint in AN, with the aim of further clarifying a model of appetite restraint to improve treatment interventions.

Keywords: RDoC, cognitive systems, anorexia nervosa, appetite restraint, impulsivity, compulsivity

1. Introduction

The Diagnostic and Statistical Manual version 5 (DSM-5), published in 2013 after a decade of edition 4, has progressed nomenclature for the psychiatric eating disorder anorexia nervosa (AN), according to three main criteria, focusing on the behaviours and cognitions underlying weight restriction and body perception [1]. Moreover, while continuing to be categorical in scope, the DSM-5 also recognises the transdiagnostic nature of AN, with the inclusion of body mass index (BMI) severity clauses: mild, moderate, severe and extreme. The BMI severity inclusion incorporates the overlapping impulsive and compulsive facets of weight dysregulation in eating disorders. For example, compulsive energy restriction relative to body weight requirements is an important diagnostic feature of AN, as is the intense fear of weight gain, and persistence in behaviour that interferes with weight gain. The third criterion includes disturbance in body perception, with undue influence of self-evaluation and persistent denial of the seriousness of reduced body weight. Restrictive and binge-purge are two subtype classifications of AN determined over the course of 3 months. The former holds if an individual has achieved weight loss by compulsive dieting, fasting or excessive exercise; the latter holds if an individual has engaged in impulsive binge-purge behaviour, including the use of diuretics, enemas, laxatives or self-induced vomiting.

The fifth edition of DSM further clarifies eating disorders and their underlying impulsive and compulsive features, incorporating additional categories such as avoidant/restrictive food intake disorder, rumination disorder, pica (compulsive consumption of non-nutritional substances) and binge eating disorder [2]. In terms of AN in particular, the behavioural (e.g. weight dysregulation) and cognitive (e.g. inflexible thinking and misperception) traits are significantly linked to genetic and environmental vulnerabilities, and more recently, to alterations in brain structure and function, particularly within the hypothalamus, hippocampus, insular cortex, parietal cortex and prefrontal cortex [3]. Furthermore, neuroinflammatory processes that contribute to the "leaky gut-brain" hypothesis of eating disorders may interact with these brain regions, via over-expression of cytokines, such as leukotrienes. Recently, theories about the involvement of neuroinflammatory processes in AN may bridge the gap between genetic susceptibility, environmental causes and changes in brain function, especially with regard to altered hypothalamic leptin and serotonin function. Moreover, memory and evaluative processes associated with dysfunction in the hippocampus and prefrontal cortex may contribute to the compulsive overvaluation of thinness, body dissatisfaction and excessive appetite restriction in AN [4], whereas the link to binge eating appears to overlap with striatal dysfunction and impulsivity [5].

The current understanding of eating disorders in general, and of AN in particular, reflects a view that impulsivity and compulsivity are significant diagnostic personality facets underlying the disorder [6]. While some propose that impulsivity and compulsivity are opposite extremes of a single personality dimension, others view impulsivity as a trait vulnerability that drives compulsivity, with repetitive behaviours that emerge as maladaptive, coping strategies to regulate arousal [7]. In addition, while both impulsive and compulsive traits appear to map onto binge eating, persistent drive for thinness and appetite restraint, with some fluctuation between these conditions [3], research suggests that impulsivity and compulsivity are entirely separate constructs that can present, to varying degrees, in unison [6]. Thus, there is still debate in the eating disorders field as to how impulsivity and compulsivity interact and correspond to the DSM criteria. In an attempt to better understand the roles, and to consider potential mechanisms, here we take the *cognitive systems* RDoC domain and its measurement, to examine the presentation of impulsivity and compulsivity and the link to cognitive processes underlying appetite restraint in AN. Prior to the examination of the RDoC domain and its measurement, next follows a brief summary of the definitions of impulsivity and compulsivity.

2. Impulsivity and compulsivity

Traditional views posit that impulsivity and compulsivity are dissociable states, reflecting neural processes within corticolimbic circuitry that underlie high arousal and maladaptive aversion avoidance, respectively [8, 9]. However, with the advancement of neuroimaging data within transdiagnostic phenotypes, influenced in part by the updated DSM-5 nomenclature in 2013, and the publication of the RDoC, there appears to be common corticolimbic neural functions that when activated in a certain pattern, correspond to high levels of automaticity, impaired cognitive inhibition, lack of self-control and maladaptive self-regulation [10]. It remains to be elucidated, however, why certain variations in impulsivity and compulsivity present as discrete types of psychiatric disorder. In addition, while common psychiatric comorbidities exist between disorders, as highlighted by the RDoC enterprise, the DSM clearly demonstrates discrete boundaries that also exist between various phenotypes. Thus, examining impulsivity and compulsivity from the transdiagnostic measurement of the RDoC cognitive systems domain may clarify how these constructs merge to form a diagnosis of restrictive or binge purge AN.

2.1 Definitions of impulsivity

The International Society for Research on Impulsivity (ISRI: http://www.impulsivity.org) defines impulsivity as: *behaviours or tendencies to act with less forethought than do most individuals of equal ability and knowledge, or a predisposition towards rapid, unplanned reactions to internal or external stimuli without regard to the negative consequences of these reactions*. Research defines impulsivity broadly as part of a normal range of functioning (as opposed to compulsivity that may reflect a maladaptive coping strategy), and yet it is the frequency of impulsivity that determines whether disorder exists [7, 11]. Moreover, neuropsychological research over the last decade has clarified the multi-faceted nature of impulsivity and its neural correlates [11] that are broadly associated with inattention or narrow/inflexible thinking (cognitive impulsivity) and hyperactivity (behavioural or motor impulsivity). Within these broad definitions, nuances of impulsivity occur [11], highlighted by research studies that deserve additional consideration. For example, choice versus rapid response impulsivity have been identified; the former concerns the preference for immediate over delayed rewards (e.g. temporal or delay discounting), the latter concerns the tendency to act without forethought and out of context with immediate demands [12, 13]. Further distinctions of impulsivity within choice versus response impulsivity have been developed [9]. For example, motor impulsivity reflects an inability to inhibit an inappropriate or misplaced response. Disadvantageous decision-making involves cognitions that underlie risk-taking behaviours, and an inability to avoid danger, threat or some form of personal loss. Choice impulsivity determines a person, who cannot delay the experience of reward (e.g. temporal or delay discounting). Finally, reflection impulsivity refers to an inability to deliberate on the potential outcome of one's actions.

2.2 Definitions of compulsivity

Impulsivity appears related to a natural, arousal response, with some adaptive qualities that are widely researched and effectively defined [11], whereas conversely, there is a lack of consensus about compulsivity – both in terms of its definition and function. However, deficits in attention, perception and repetition of motor or cognitive responses appear to be key facets [9]. A recent formal definition based on neuroscientific research states that compulsivity is *a tendency towards repetitive, habitual actions, repeated despite adverse consequences* [14]. Compulsive, perpetual and ritualised behaviours and cognitions may be attempts to neutralise high levels of arousal and negative affect (e.g., fear, anxiety and perceived threat) and for the individual to gain a rewarding sense of control. However, in recent years, there have been various attempts to better conceptualise the nuances of compulsivity, and to date four discrete definitions have been emerged [9]. First, contingency-related cognitive inflexibility refers to heightened perseverance, especially in anticipation of receipt of a previously experienced reward. Second, task/attentional set-shifting deficits refer to an inability to alter cognitive strategies as the task/attentional demands change. Third, attentional bias/disengagement concerns the phenomenon of disorder salience, where certain stimuli bias processing resources, which may delay the completion of concurrent cognitive tasks (e.g. the "Food Stroop" task for eating disorders [15]). Finally, habit learning describes repetitive automaticity of behaviours and cognitions that correspond to a previously experienced reward.

2.3 Interactions between impulsivity and compulsivity

A diathesis model has held for many years, whereby the constructs of impulsivity and compulsivity are at opposing ends of a spectrum [9]. Such a model suggests that compulsive, maladaptive coping strategies manage excessively impulsive, automatic arousal reactions to internal and external stimuli. In support of the diathesis model, the Pavlovian Instrumental Transfer (PIT) theory [16] describes a switch from deliberative, controlled, ventral striatal (nucleus accumbens-driven) activation to habitual, repetitive, uncontrolled, dorsal striatal (caudate, putamen-driven) activation associated with reward. Furthermore, psychiatric compulsive cognitions and behaviours may be attempts to reduce high levels of impulsivity, arousal, tension and negative affect [8]. In this vein, trait vulnerability for high levels of impulsivity is associated with the advent and maintenance of psychiatric disorder, whereas the role of compulsivity is less clear, but may provide the individual with a semblance of respite from psychological distress, which is rewarding from an opponent process perspective [17]. Support for this notion comes from the repetitive nature of compulsivity – in that, an element of reward must be present for a cognition or behaviour to be repeated. Furthermore, by repeating the process of tension/stress reduction, an allostatic load alteration occurs to maintain stability within neural circuits, which ultimately contributes to psychiatric disorder [18]. Interestingly, the allostatic load hypothesis of AN is related to changes in basal ganglia dopaminergic and hypothalamic pituitary adrenal (HPA) axis systems [19] that are influenced by elevated inflammatory molecules (e.g. leukotrienes).

3. Impulsivity and compulsivity in AN

Impulsivity is typically associated with the loss-of-control over eating, which is characteristic of the binge-purge AN subtype, bulimia nervosa and binge eating disorder [20]. In contrast, the restrictive AN subtype is associated with disproportionate belief systems about self-control (e.g. preferring the goal of future thinness to present eating), whereas binge eating subtypes have steeper delay discounting rates and disinhibition over rapid eating [20]. Additionally, higher levels of impulsivity in those with bingeing subtypes of eating disorder show lower goal-drive persistence [21]. Interestingly, the bingeing subtypes, including binge-purge AN, also tend to present with other impulse control disorders, such as gambling disorder, which have a higher preponderance for impulsivity, suicidality and cognitive distortions [22]. Higher levels of impulsivity in binge-purge AN subtypes also correspond to increased difficulties in emotion regulation that may worsen with older age [23]. Finally, perhaps most pertinent to the role of impulsivity in bingeing subtypes of eating disorder is the concept of negative urgency, which is the dispositional tendency to engage in rash action during the experience of negative affect. Women with AN, who score higher on negative urgency, with an experience of negative affect, are significantly more likely to engage in binge eating behaviour [24]. Thus, in the same vein that trait vulnerability for impulsivity underlies a switch from deliberative to compulsive drug taking [25], it might be that a similar vulnerability occurs in AN, underlying a switch – or fluctuation – between impulsive binge eating and compulsive appetite restraint.

Compulsivity in AN refers to the relentless pursuit of appetite restraint and weight loss, which appears to be transdiagnostic and related to obsessive-compulsive and addictive disorders [26]. In fact, obsessive-compulsive personality disorder, and addictive processes are common comorbidities in restrictive AN, alongside anxiety and depression [27, 28]. The compulsive relationship between initially rewarding deliberative behaviours and the relentless pursuit of thinness, supported by excessive exercise, starvation and purging, is associated with aberrant cortico-striatal dysfunction and rigid, inflexible cognitive ruminations [25]. Moreover, the physiological effects of excessive weight loss may encourage the development of compulsive traits by altering neuroinflammatory processes within the gut-brain axis that interfere with memory consolidation physiology in the hippocampus and prefrontal cortex, and appetite dysregulation in the hypothalamus. A neural shift within corticolimbic brain areas underlying compulsive behaviour may explain why not all people who experiment with illicit substances become addicted, and not all people who experiment with dieting develop an eating disorder. However, the switch to a compulsive pursuit of thinness and appetite restraint in AN appears rewarding similar to the addictive process [28]. The cause of the switch to compulsive behaviour is not yet elucidated. However, it encompasses trait vulnerability for anxiety and impulsivity, and an initial controlled experience of reward (e.g. the pleasure of self-control and social praise alongside dieting), the development of incentive salience to motivate the continuance of the behaviour, and finally the seeking, or habitual behaviour necessary to repeat the learned reward [29]. Additionally, aberrant opponent processes in corticolimbic circuitry underlying reward deficits and stress surfeits drive compulsivity [29], which for those with AN would mean increasingly dangerous, yet still rewarding, weight loss attempts.

3.1 Multi-faceted elements of impulsivity and compulsivity in AN

Impulsivity and compulsivity may both uniquely contribute, in varying degrees, to certain aspects of AN. Compelling evidence suggests that both facets of impulsivity and compulsivity contribute to eating concerns and restraint in AN [6]. In a recent study of adults with AN by Lavender and colleagues [6], extensive self-report measures were used to confirm that impulsivity was linked to eating concerns and the frequency of loss of control eating. Conversely, compulsivity was associated with the lack of perseverance and restraint, as well as eating and weight concerns. Previously, the RDoC criteria reinforce the notion that anxiety drives the compulsive tendency to engage in repetitive self-starvation in those with AN [28]. This is in line with recent suggestions that impulsivity is associated with heightened anxiety, or negative urgency, which appears to drive maladaptive compulsive strategies in those with eating disorders [30]. **Figure 1** provides a schematic diagram of the link between arousal, anxiety, binge eating, restraint, impulsivity and compulsivity in AN.

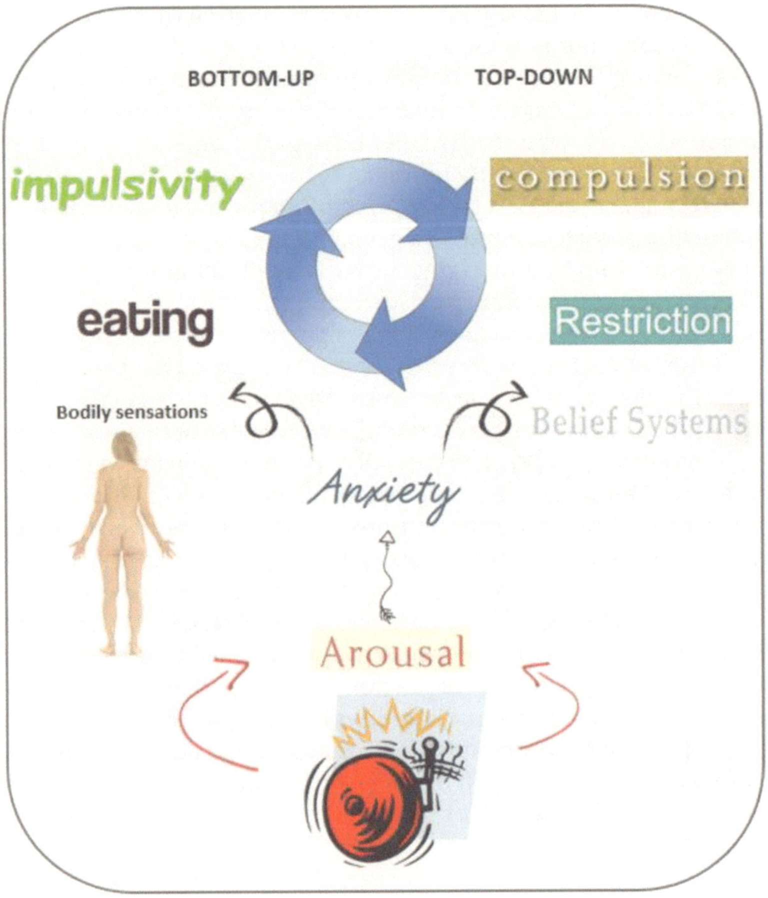

Figure 1.
A schematic diagram describing how impulsivity and compulsivity may interact with bodily sensations (bottom up) and belief systems (top-down) in binge-eating and restricting anorexia nervosa (AN).

4. The RDoC research domains and suggested units of measurement

Some consensus appears in the eating disorder literature as to the role of impulsivity and compulsivity in binge eating and restrictive eating subtypes, respectively. However, there is still debate as to whether these are separate constructs, extremes on a diathesis model, or functioning concomitantly in varying degrees to derive a fluctuating eating disorder phenotype. Moreover, there are other nuances to eating disorders – such as body and self-image distortion, denial of disorder, cognitive deficits including excessive attention to detail, set-shifting abnormalities – that are still not fully elucidated by theories of the neural processes of impulsivity and compulsivity. As such, it is useful to consider the transdiagnostic scope of the RDoC domains and suggested units of measurement, in an attempt to further clarify how impulsivity and compulsivity might contribute to symptoms of the subtypes of AN.

4.1 Five RDoC domains

RDoC comprises of five domains for suggested neuroscientific research areas (see: https://www.nimh.nih.gov/research-priorities/rdoc/constructs/rdoc-matrix.shtml). These are: (i) negative valence systems; (ii) positive valence systems; (iii) cognitive systems; (iv) social processes and (v) arousal and regulatory systems.

Negative valence systems include fear, anxiety, sustained threat, loss and frustrative non-reward. Positive valence systems include reward responsiveness, reward learning and reward valuation. Cognitive systems include attention, perception, declarative memory, language, cognitive control and working memory. Social processes include attachment, social communication, perception and understanding of the self, perception and understanding of others. Finally, arousal and regulatory systems include circadian rhythms and sleep/wakefulness. Against the background of the RDoC domains, given the scope of this article, the cognitive systems domain, linking impulsivity and compulsivity to varying degrees of appetite restraint in AN, will be the focus of the remaining sections.

4.2 Eight RDoC measures

To measure the cognitive systems domain, the RDoC suggests eight neuroscientific genres. These are: (i) genes; (ii) molecules (neurotransmitters); (iii) cells; (iv) neural circuits; (v) physiology; (vi) behaviour; (vii) self-report; and (viii) paradigms. Before considering how cognitive systems and their measurement might aid the understanding of the role of impulsivity and compulsivity in appetite-restraint variations characteristic of AN, the measurement of the cognitive systems domain will be defined below. As a brief introduction, attention may be related to cognitive biases (particularly toward food and body-image stimuli) that maintain cognitive restraint in AN. Perception can be linked to non-conscious sensory mechanisms that may drive maladaptive conscious evaluations of the environment in those with AN. Declarative memories may underlie the AN narrative of the self and the world. Language processing may support the development of the internal narrative associated with AN-related cognitions, particularly in line with becoming and staying thin and in control. Cognitive control refers to the ability of people with AN to excessively regulate their appetite and eating behaviours with cognitive ruminations of goals to stay underweight. Finally, working memory likely underpins the flexible updating of excessively detailed cognitive strategies to achieve the future goal of thinness, and to avoid immediate distractions (e.g. food-related stimuli). Next follows a detailed account of the RDoC definitions of the sub-constructs (attention, perception, declarative memory, language, cognitive control and working memory) and the measurement of the cognitive systems domain.

4.2.1 Attention

According to the RDoC, attention refers to the regulation of capacity-limited systems such as awareness, higher order perception and motor function (e.g. response inhibition). Additionally, the RDoC clarifies that capacity limitation and competition are synonymous with selective and divided attention, respectively, which relate to attentional bias and distraction. The measurement of genes associated with attention has yielded inconclusive findings. However, in terms of neurotransmitters, the RDoC highlights that a balance between GABAergic and glutamatergic systems within the prefrontal cortex is a key to implement attention. Specifically, the control of attention is associated with acetylcholine, dopamine, glutamate, histamine and serotonin. In terms of cells, the RDoC recognises parvalbumin-positive interneurons as linked to the process of attention. Brain circuits associated with the initiation of attention include a balance between the resting state default mode and task positive networks, whereas the subsequent control of attention links to descending and ascending networks with the corticolimbic circuitry. Additionally, the dorsal "where" and ventral "what" visual processing pathways are implicated in attentional neural networks. Physiological measures of attention have yielded most consistent results according to the RDoC, with functional MRI (fMRI), auditory/visual event-related potentials (ERPs) and peripheral measures such as heart rate and pupillometry. The RDoC goes on to list that behavioural measures associated with attention include task distractibility, attentional lapses versus sustained attention, distractibility, object/feature detection, psychophysics and spatial attention. Finally, in terms of paradigms that measure attention, these include attentional blink, dichotic listening, dual-task paradigms, cueing paradigms, time-series responses and visual search.

4.2.2 Perception

Perception is the process by which computations in the brain extract sensory information to construct a model of the environment, making predictions about the world and guiding action, according to the RDoC. Visual and auditory perception involves various neurotransmitter systems, such as acetylcholine, catecholamines, GABA, glutamate, NMDA, peptides and serotonin. The cells involved in visual perception are magno and parvo cells, parvalbumin-positive interneurons and pyramidal cells, whereas for auditory perception, the cells include cochlear hair cells, cortical and limbic interneurons and ribbon synapses. In terms of neural circuits, subcortical vision involves konio-, magno- and parvo-cells, cortically the supra- and infra-granular layers are involved, and also the dorsal and ventral visual streams. Additionally, the suprachiasmatic nucleus and superior colliculus control saccadic and other visual actions. Additionally, auditory perception includes brain regions such as the anterior insula, brainstem, cochlear, inferior colliculus and the superior temporal gyrus. In terms of physiology, adaption and habituation are measured via fMRI, EEG and ERPs. Behavioural experiments to incorporate visual and auditory perception include discrimination, identification and localisation, learning, priming, reading, stimulus detection and visual acuity. Commonly used paradigms in visual perception research include backward masking (subliminal processing), motion processing, contrast sensitivity, emotion expression identification, face identification, object recognition, reading and visual illusion susceptibility. Commonly used paradigms in auditory perception research include auditory masking, streaming, detection of speech in noise, gating, inhibitory control, the McGurk effect (multisensory), oddball detection, self-monitoring and tone detection. Additionally, olfactory research is an emerging area of interest, with different odours eliciting different perceptual and cognitive systems.

4.2.3 Declarative memory

Declarative memory refers to the acquisition, encoding, storage and retrieval of information gained from the environment. This type of memory, as opposed to non-conscious, non-declarative memory, is important for spatial, temporal and contextual information, which represents a timeframe of events (e.g. episodic), and the organisation of items of memories into facts (semantic). Inferential and flexible extraction occurs from memories in order to update novel sensory information (e.g. Bayesian Inference). According to the RDoC, the neurotransmitters involved in declarative memory include acetylcholine, glutamate, noradrenalin and opioids. In terms on neuronal cell types that support declarative memory, these are glia, granule cells, inhibitory and excitatory interneurons and pyramidal cells. Brain circuitry for memory involves the hippocampus, and connections between the prefrontal and parietal cortices, as well as various other association areas. The physiology that supports declarative memory includes AMPA-related synaptic plasticity, coordinated fronto-temporal oscillatory activity, long-term potentiation and long-term depression and changes in the fMRI, EEG or other spatial and temporal brain imaging measures. Behaviour associated with declarative memory is measured by discrimination and familiarity tests, or learning, recall and recognition tasks. Finally, various paradigms exist to test declarative memory, including delayed recall, acquired equivalence, list and story learning, paired associative learning and transitive inference.

4.2.4 Language

The RDoC describes cognitive processes underlying language as a system of shared symbolic representations of the external environment, incorporating abstract and self-related notions that aid thought and communication. Currently, there are no conclusive data regarding the genes, neurotransmitters or cells that contribute to language. However, the neural circuitry involves the inferior fronto-temporo-parietal cortices, superior and middle temporal cortices, with considerable involvement of the limbic system, motor and sensory cortices. Behaviour is measured in the form of coherent discourse and sentences, and incorporates Wernicke (temporal cortex) and Broca's (frontal cortex) areas for speech comprehension and production, respectively. Experimental paradigms include discourse analyses and eye-tracking equipment.

4.2.5 Cognitive control

The RDoC defines cognitive control as the processes that modulate the operation of other cognitive and affective systems in the brain. Cognitive control processes enable the achievement of goal-oriented behaviour, when pre-potent responses are not adequate for current demands. Control processes are also important under conditions of uncertainty, or novelty, where appropriate responses are selected from various competing options. Cognitive control involves three sub-processes, according to the RDoC: goal selection (updating, representation and maintenance), response selection (inhibition/suppression), and performance monitoring. Firstly, goal selection involves dorsolateral prefrontal and parietal cortex function, as well as inhibition of the default mode network. The neurotransmitter systems involved include cholinergic, dopaminergic, GABAergic, glutamatergic and norepinephrine. Gamma synchrony and pupillometry are some physiological measures used to detect goal-oriented cognitive control, alongside behavioural measures of distractibility. Experimental paradigms include cued stimulus-response reversal tasks, task switching and tower tasks (e.g. Hanoi, London). In addition, response selection tasks measure impulsive behaviour, using paradigms such as the Flanker, Simon and Stroop tests. Furthermore, response inhibition typically involves the parietal cortex, pre-supplementary motor area and ventro-fronto-striatal circuitry. Physiology of response inhibition is probed using, for example, pupillometry, eye-blink startle paradigms and transcranial magnetic stimulation. Tasks associated with response inhibition include Go/No-Go and Stop-Signal Reaction Time tasks. Finally, performance monitoring appears to involve serotonergic and dopaminergic systems within the anterior cingulate cortex, pre-supplementary motor area and insula and measured by conflict monitoring tasks.

4.2.6 Working memory

The RDoC definition states that working memory is active maintenance and flexible updating of goal or task relevant information (e.g. holding in mind bits of information, strategies and plans) in a limited capacity store that resists interference. This active maintenance could involve flexible binding together of bits of information, may be internally represented despite external cues and holding in mind may be temporary, although this could be a function of interference. As such, according to the RDoC, working memory constitutes four sub-components: active maintenance, flexible updating, limited capacity and interference control. Active maintenance involves D1 dopamine receptor function, dopamine, GABA, glutamate and NMDA within inhibitory and pyramidal neuron populations. Furthermore, the cells responsible for inhibitory control include calbindin, calretinin, parvalbumin and distinct types of inhibitory neurons. Neural circuitry for active maintenance includes dorsolateral and ventrolateral prefrontal-parietal cortex and cingulate-thalamo-limbic networks. Additionally, medium spiny neurons in the basal ganglia enable flexible updating. Delta, theta and gamma waves are also implicated with the use of EEG recordings. Working memory cognitive paradigms include change detection tasks, complex span tasks, delayed match to sample and non-sample, letter-number sequencing, N-Back, self-ordered pointing, sequence encoding and reproduction and Sternberg item recognition.

4.3 RDoC measures of cognitive systems and the role of impulsivity and compulsivity in AN

See **Table 1** for the summary of the RDoC cognitive systems sub-domains and their link to impulsivity and compulsivity in AN. The RDoC cognitive systems domain includes the constructs attention, perception, declarative memory, language, cognitive control and working memory, and all are pertinent in the processes of appetite control in AN. Before considering the RDoC measures of these constructs in relation to AN phenotypes, the broad links to these constructs are summarised. First, attentional processes are associated with regulatory control and response inhibition, and underlie the conscious and non-conscious processes of attentional bias to food stimuli [15, 31]. For example, attention is influenced by incentive salience as reflected in eye-blink startle responses to disorder-specific cues [32], which could drive the cognitive tendency for delayed reporting of disorder-specific stimuli [15]. Second, perception is related to this, and encompasses Bayesian Inference and epistemic foraging, or in AN-related terms, excessive cognitive sampling (e.g. of internal or external stimuli), to create rigid, inflexible cognitive models about the self, world and others, especially under conditions of uncertainty [4]. Third, declarative memory links to perception, in that episodic memory for recent food consumption for example, alters semantic memory regarding the metabolic and hedonic need for food [33]. However, recent research has not been able to replicate the finding that focused attention during eating improves later appetite control, and so, more research is required to determine under what conditions attention is associated with appetite control [34]. Fourth, language processes may support the internal narrative that contributes to ruminations underlying a distorted view of self and of body image [35]. Cognitive control may explain the compulsive nature of cognitive ruminations in AN, which bias decision-making and contribute to affect dysregulation [36]. Fifth, cognitive control of appetite may involve either goal-oriented cognitive inhibition of distracting stimuli, or pre-potent motor response inhibition [33]. Finally, working memory may contribute to the cognitive control of appetite by keeping in mind, for delayed periods, independent of the initial stimulus (e.g. food), detailed and complex strategies to avoid eating [4]. Next follows a more detailed account of how the RDoC measures of cognitive systems might contribute to an updated understanding of the role of impulsivity and compulsivity in AN.

4.3.1 Impulsivity

Binge-eating AN phenotypes are typically associated with trait impulsivity [5, 8, 9]. As such, the level of distraction (by food or body images for example) caused attention, as well as deficits in response inhibition (e.g. go/no-go, Stop Signal tasks and pre-pulse inhibition tasks), is likely to be a predictor of disorder severity reflected in distinct neural functioning [37]. Specifically, the function of acetylcholine, dopamine, glutamate, histamine and serotonin, and related stress hormones, particularly in the prefrontal-basal ganglia circuitry, are likely to be significantly indicative of the degree of impulsivity, and the likelihood that a binge-eating AN phenotype is present [38]. Similarly, neuronal variability in the ventral attentional resting state network may well reflect a greater propensity for impulsivity, and deficits in appetite control [39]. Heart rate variability and pupillometry may also highlight non-consciously derived arousal subserving impulsive tendencies and the binge-eating subtypes [40, 41].

4.3.2 Compulsivity

Restrictive subtypes of AN are typically associated with compulsivity, for example, inflexible ruminations and excessive attention to detail that appear to regulate anxiety and maintain complex self-concepts about weight loss [35]. Moreover, altered perceptual processes are associated with specific central coherence and empathy deficits, such as an inability to perceive a global view [42], read the mind in the eyes [43] and alexithymia–an inability to recognise one's own or others' internal states [44]. Ineffective affect regulation, particularly in terms of anxiety and depression, may drive the compulsive tendency to rely on cognitive evaluations for environmental navigation and decision-making in those with restrictive AN [4]. Furthermore, studies of subliminal priming demonstrate that restrictive AN patients, particularly those with high levels of anxiety, experience

RDoC cognitive systems sub-domain with definition	Measures of impulsivity	Measures of compulsivity
Attention: *The regulation of capacity-limited systems such as awareness, higher-order perception and motor function (e.g. response inhibition).*	Binge-purge severity is significantly associated with impulsivity, and is predicted by the level of distraction (by food or body images for example) caused to attention, as well as deficits in response inhibition (e.g. go/no-go, Stop Signal tasks and pre-pulse inhibition tasks). This is reflected in distinct neural functioning within fronto-striatal circuitry [37]. Acetylcholine, dopamine, glutamate, histamine and serotonin function, and related stress hormones, particularly in the prefrontal-basal ganglia circuitry, are related to the degree of impulsivity, and the likelihood that a binge-eating AN phenotype is present [38].	Restrictive subtypes of AN are typically associated with compulsivity, for example, inflexible obsessive-compulsive ruminations and excessive attention to detail that appear to regulate anxiety and maintain complex self-concepts about weight loss [35]. An imbalance between GABAergic and glutamatergic systems within the prefrontal cortex is key to the compulsive function of attention (e.g. towards food and body stimuli) in AN. Task distractibility, attentional lapses versus sustained attention, distractibility, object/feature detection, psychophysics and spatial attention are common cognitive tasks used to measure attentional compulsivity.

RDoC cognitive systems sub-domain with definition	Measures of impulsivity	Measures of compulsivity
Perception: *The process by which computations in the brain extract sensory information to construct a model of the environment, making predictions about the world and guiding action.*	Heart-rate variability and pupillometry may highlight non-consciously derived perceptual processes sub-serving impulsive tendencies and the binge-eating subtypes [40, 41]. The dorsal 'where' and ventral 'what' visual processing pathways are implicated in rapid responses to environmental stimuli. Backward masking (subliminal processing), motion processing, contrast sensitivity, emotion expression identification, face identification, object recognition, reading, and visual illusion susceptibility. See also the McGurk effect (multisensory), oddball detection, self-monitoring and tone detection.	Altered perceptual processes are associated with specific central coherence and empathy deficits, such as an inability to perceive a global view [42], read the mind in the eyes [43] and alexithymia - an inefficiency in perceiving one's own or others' internal states [44]. A switch from deliberative dieting to compulsive appetite restriction may involve a switch from activation of incentive salience networks within nucleus accumbens systems in favour of dorsal striatum networks associated with Pavlovian Instrumental Transfer [25]. The suprachiasmatic nucleus and superior colliculus control saccadic and other visual actions associated with excessive epistemic foraging of the environment, measured by eye-tracking equipment.
Declarative memory: *The acquisition, encoding, storage and retrieval of information gained from the environment.*	Declarative memory is important for spatial, temporal and contextual information, which represents a timeframe of events (e.g. episodic), and the organisation of items of memories into facts (semantic). Inferential and flexible extraction occurs from memories in order to update novel sensory information (e.g. Bayesian Inference). This may underlie conditioned fear and threat-related impulsive responses to food, eating and the environment. Fluctuating levels of acetylcholine, glutamate, noradrenalin and opioids. In terms on neuronal cell types that support declarative memory, these are glia, granule cells, inhibitory and excitatory interneurons and pyramidal cells.	Compulsive cognitive ruminations and biases, which reflect in eye-tracking studies of vigilance and avoidance [46] may therefore become more deeply conditioned and consolidated in connected regions such as hippocampal, prefrontal cortex, and cholinergic and striatal dopaminergic neurons [47]. This may alter non-conscious memory formation and increase the probability of cognitive biases to disorder-relevant stimuli [48].
Language: *A system of shared symbolic representations of the external environment, incorporating abstract and self-related notions that aid thought and communication.*	Inferior fronto-temporo-parietal cortices, superior and middle temporal cortices, with considerable involvement of the limbic system, motor and sensory cortices. This may underlie the negative self-talk and phonological loop activation associated with impulsive responses to perceived threat and subsequent binge eating, which acts as a maladaptive coping strategy to suppress negative affect.	Coherent discourse analysis, which is reflected in neural function of Wernicke (temporal cortex) and Broca's (frontal cortex) areas for speech comprehension and production, respectively could measure restrictive eating behaviour that may be driven by cognitive ruminations. Experimental paradigms include discourse analyses and eye-tracking equipment.

RDoC cognitive systems sub-domain with definition	Measures of impulsivity	Measures of compulsivity
Cognitive control: *The processes that modulate the operation of other cognitive and affective systems in the brain. Cognitive control processes enable the achievement of goal-oriented behaviour, when pre-potent responses are not adequate for current demands.*	Neuronal variability in the ventral attentional resting state network may well reflect a greater propensity for impulsivity, and deficits in appetite control [39]. Varying levels of control of attention is associated with levels of fluctuating acetylcholine, dopamine, glutamate, histamine and serotonin. Parvalbumin-positive interneurons are linked to the process of attentional control.	Ineffective affect regulation, particularly in terms of anxiety and depression, may drive the compulsive tendency to rely on cognitive evaluations for environmental navigation and decision-making in those with restrictive AN [4]. A discrete balance between GABAergic and glutamatergic neurotransmitter function in the prefrontal cortex may underpin excessive cognitive control of appetite in restrictive AN, and superior performance on planning tasks [4].
Working memory: *The active maintenance and flexible updating of goal or task relevant information (e.g. holding in mind bits of information, strategies, and plans) in a limited capacity store that resists interference.*	A balance between the resting state default mode and task positive networks underlies the maintenance of working memory and the subsequent control of attention links to descending and ascending networks with the corticolimbic and parietal cortex circuitry.	Studies of subliminal priming (with food images for e.g.) demonstrate that restrictive AN patients, particularly those with high levels of anxiety, experience the greatest interference to cognitive processes such as working memory [31, 45]. Greater working memory capacity may in turn contribute to the holding in mind of excessively detailed cognitive ruminations (e.g. epistemic foraging) in the absence of food stimuli, which subsequently resists interference (e.g. from interoceptive or exteroceptive stimuli).

Table 1.
RDoC cognitive systems sub-domain definitions and measures of impulsivity and compulsivity in relation to anorexia nervosa (binge-purge and restraint subtypes).

interference to cognitive processes, such as working memory [31, 45]. Greater working memory capacity may in turn contribute to the holding in mind of excessively detailed cognitive ruminations in the absence of food stimuli. As such, a discrete balance between GABAergic and glutamatergic neurotransmitter function in the prefrontal cortex may underpin excessive cognitive control of appetite in restrictive AN, and superior performance on working memory and planning tasks [4]. Moreover, a switch from deliberative dieting to compulsive appetite restriction may involve a switch from activation of incentive salience networks within nucleus accumbens systems in favour of dorsal striatum networks associated with Pavlovian Instrumental Transfer [25]. Compulsive cognitive ruminations and biases, which reflect in eye-tracking studies of vigilance and avoidance [46] may therefore become more deeply engrained and consolidated in connected regions such as hippocampal, cholinergic and striatal dopaminergic neurons [47]. This may alter non-conscious memory formation and increase the probability of cognitive biases to disorder-relevant stimuli [48]. Finally, a propensity to higher levels of anxiety is associated with compulsive ruminations in AN, as well as the common presentation of obsessive-compulsive and other psychiatric disorders [49].

5. Conclusions

Considering the facets of impulsivity and compulsivity in AN from the perspective of the cognitive systems, RDoC domain may aid understanding of the nuances of appetite control in eating disorders. Traditionally, impulsivity is associated with binge-eating subtypes, which incorporates response inhibition deficits, craving, errors of perception, deficits in affect regulation and decision-making. In contrast, compulsivity appears to underlie the drive for thinness and excessive cognitive ruminations about food, eating, shape and weight concerns, and the control of eating in restrictive AN. As such, attention, declarative memory systems, perceptual processes, language and internal narratives, cognitive control processes and working memory–to hold consciously in mind complex strategies and detailed plans–appear significantly associated with restrictive AN. Moreover, heightened anxiety and altered incentive salience, non-consciously represented by mesolimbic function, appear to drive the compulsive maladaptive coping strategies. Thus, impulsivity and compulsivity may not form a diathesis model in AN, but they may rather overlap. Given this potential overlap, it might be that treatment interventions effectively treat one and not the other, which could form a basis for relapse. For example, altering maladaptive, compulsive cognitions during cognitive-behavioural therapy treatment without sufficiently altering impulsive, non-consciously-derived appetitive arousal and anxiety (to food or body images, for example), could drive the eventual re-emergence of maladaptive cognitions and relapse.

The popularity and relative efficacy of cognitive behavioural therapy for eating disorders may be due, in part, to the effective measurement of conscious, compulsive restraint cognitions – with self-report or neurocognitive paradigms for example – that may be easier to measure than non-consciously derived impulsive tendencies. Despite this, standard treatments for eating disorders continue to be subject to high relapse rates. However, the RD0C provides suggestions for other measures, such as cellular systems, genes, molecules (neurotransmitters) and neural systems that may well influence conscious compulsions, but are themselves functioning non-consciously within biological systems. With this in mind, measures of impulsivity (e.g. anxiety, appetitive and non-conscious responses to food) may help to inform treatment efficacy, alongside more deliberative, psychological measures of compulsivity (e.g. self-report, neurocognitive tasks). Measuring the overlap between impulsivity and compulsivity in AN, from the perspective of the RDoC cognitive systems domain, may enable a more accurate model of appetite restraint that can improve relapse rates post-treatment.

Conflict of interest

The author declares no conflict of interest.

Author details

Samantha Jane Brooks[1*] and Helgi Schiöth[2]

1 School of Natural Sciences and Psychology, Liverpool John Moores University, Liverpool, United Kingdom

2 Head of Section of Functional Pharmacology, Department of Neuroscience, Uppsala University, BMC, Uppsala, Sweden

*Address all correspondence to: s.j.brooks@ljmu.ac.uk

References

[1] First MB. Diagnostic and statistical manual of mental disorders, 5th edition, and clinical utility. The Journal of Nervous and Mental Disease. 2013;**201**(9):727-729

[2] Call C, Walsh BT, Attia E. From DSM-IV to DSM-5: Changes to eating disorder diagnoses. Current Opinion in Psychiatry. 2013;**26**(6):532-536

[3] Treasure J, Zipfel S, Micali N, Wade T, Stice E, Claudino A, et al. Anorexia nervosa. Nature Reviews Disease Primers. 2015;**1**:15074

[4] Brooks SJ, Funk SG, Young SY, Schioth HB. The role of working memory for cognitive control in anorexia nervosa versus substance use disorder. Frontiers in Psychology. 2017;**8**:1651

[5] Collier DA, Treasure JL. The aetiology of eating disorders. The British Journal of Psychiatry. 2004;**185**:363-365

[6] Lavender JM, Goodman EL, Culbert KM, Wonderlich SA, Crosby RD, Engel SG, et al. Facets of impulsivity and compulsivity in women with anorexia nervosa. European Eating Disorders Review. 2017;**25**(4):309-313

[7] Brooks SJ, Lochner C, Shoptaw S, Stein DJ. Using the research domain criteria (RDoC) to conceptualize impulsivity and compulsivity in relation to addiction. Progress in Brain Research. 2017;**235**:177-218

[8] Dalley JW, Everitt BJ, Robbins TW. Impulsivity, compulsivity, and top-down cognitive control. Neuron. 2011;**69**(4):680-694

[9] Fineberg NA, Chamberlain SR, Goudriaan AE, Stein DJ, Vanderschuren LJ, Gillan CM, et al. New developments in human neurocognition: Clinical, genetic, and brain imaging correlates of impulsivity and compulsivity. CNS Spectrums. 2014;**19**(1):69-89

[10] Brooks SJ, Lochner C, Shoptaw S, Stein DJ. Using the research domain criteria (RDoC) to conceptualise impulsivity and compulsivity in relation to addiction. Progress in Brain Research. 2017;**235**:177-218

[11] Dalley JW, Robbins TW. Fractionating impulsivity: Neuropsychiatric implications. Nature Reviews Neuroscience. 2017;**18**(3):158-171

[12] Hamilton KR, Littlefield AK, Anastasio NC, Cunningham KA, Fink LHL, Wing VC, et al. Rapid-response impulsivity: Definitions, measurement issues, and clinical implications. Personality Disorders: Theory, Research, and Treatment. 2015;**6**(2):168-181

[13] Hamilton KR, Mitchell MR, Wing VC, Balodis IM, Bickel WK, Fillmore M, et al. Choice impulsivity: Definitions, measurement issues, and clinical implications. Personality Disorders: Theory, Research, and Treatment. 2015;**6**(2):182-198

[14] Chamberlain SR, Stochl J, Redden SA, Grant JE. Latent traits of impulsivity and compulsivity: Toward dimensional psychiatry. Psychological Medicine. 2018;**48**(5):810-821

[15] Brooks S, Prince A, Stahl D, Campbell IC, Treasure J. A systematic review and meta-analysis of cognitive bias to food stimuli in people with disordered eating behaviour. Clinical Psychology Review. 2011;**31**(1): 37-51

[16] Cartoni E, Balleine B, Baldassarre G. Appetitive Pavlovian-instrumental transfer: A review. Neuroscience and Biobehavioral Reviews. 2016;**71**:829-848

[17] Koob GF, Le MMR. Neurobiological mechanisms for opponent motivational processes in addiction. Philosophical Transactions of the Royal Society of London. Series B, Biological Sciences. 2008;**363**(1507):3113-3123

[18] George O, Le Moal M, Koob GF. Allostasis and addiction: Role of the dopamine and corticotropin-releasing factor systems. Physiology & Behavior. 2012;**106**(1):58-64

[19] Woods SC, Begg DP. Regulation of the motivation to eat. Current Topics in Behavioral Neurosciences. 2016;**27**:15-34

[20] Steward T, Mestre-Bach G, Vintro-Alcaraz C, Aguera Z, Jimenez-Murcia S, Granero R, et al. Delay discounting of reward and impulsivity in eating disorders: From anorexia nervosa to binge eating disorder. European Eating Disorders Review. 2017;**25**(6):601-606

[21] Wilson DR, Loxton NJ, O'Shannessy D, Sheeran N, Morgan A. Similarities and differences in revised reinforcement sensitivities across eating disorder subtypes. Appetite. 2018;**133**:70-76

[22] Kim HS, von Ranson KM, Hodgins DC, McGrath DS, Tavares H. Demographic, psychiatric, and personality correlates of adults seeking treatment for disordered gambling with a comorbid binge/purge type eating disorder. European Eating Disorders Review. 2018;**26**(5):508-518

[23] Anderson LK, Claudat K, Cusack A, Brown TA, Trim J, Rockwell R, et al. Differences in emotion regulation difficulties among adults and adolescents across eating disorder diagnoses. Journal of Clinical Psychology. 2018;**74**(10):1867-1873

[24] Culbert KM, Lavender JM, Crosby RD, Wonderlich SA, Engel SG, Peterson CB, et al. Associations between negative affect and binge/purge behaviors in women with anorexia nervosa: Considering the role of negative urgency. Comprehensive Psychiatry. 2016;**66**:104-112

[25] Everitt BJ. Neural and psychological mechanisms underlying compulsive drug seeking habits and drug memories–indications for novel treatments of addiction. The European Journal of Neuroscience. 2014;**40**(1):2163-2182

[26] Godier LR, Park RJ. Compulsivity in anorexia nervosa: A transdiagnostic concept. Frontiers in Psychology. 2014;**5**:778

[27] Gillan CM, Fineberg NA, Robbins TW. A trans-diagnostic perspective on obsessive-compulsive disorder. Psychological Medicine. 2017;**47**(9):1528-1548

[28] O'Hara CB, Campbell IC, Schmidt U. A reward-centred model of anorexia nervosa: A focussed narrative review of the neurological and psychophysiological literature. Neuroscience and Biobehavioral Reviews. 2015;**52**:131-152

[29] Koob GF, Volkow ND. Neurobiology of addiction: A neurocircuitry analysis. Lancet Psychiatry. 2016;**3**(8):760-773

[30] Fischer S, Smith GT, Cyders MA. Another look at impulsivity: A meta-analytic review comparing specific dispositions to rash action in their relationship to bulimic symptoms. Clinical Psychology Review. 2008;**28**(8):1413-1425

[31] Brooks SJ, O'Daly OG, Uher R, Schioth HB, Treasure J, Campbell IC. Subliminal food images compromise superior working memory performance in women with restricting anorexia nervosa. Consciousness and Cognition. 2012;**21**(2):751-763

[32] O'Hara CB, Keyes A, Renwick B, Giel KE, Campbell IC, Schmidt U.

Evidence that illness-compatible cues are rewarding in women recovered from anorexia nervosa: A study of the effects of dopamine depletion on eye-blink startle responses. PLoS One. 2016;**11**(10):e0165104

[33] Higgs S, Spetter MS. Cognitive control of eating: The role of memory in appetite and weight gain. Current Obesity Reports. 2018;7(1):50-59

[34] Whitelock V, Higgs S, Brunstrom JM, Halford JCG, Robinson E. No effect of focused attention whilst eating on later snack food intake: Two laboratory experiments. Appetite. 2018;**128**:188-196

[35] Smith KE, Mason TB, Lavender JM. Rumination and eating disorder psychopathology: A meta-analysis. Clinical Psychology Review. 2018;**61**:9-23

[36] Danner UN, Sternheim L, Bijsterbosch JM, Dingemans AE, Evers C, van Elburg AA. Influence of negative affect on decision making in women with restrictive and binge-purge type anorexia nervosa. Psychiatry Research. 2016;**239**:39-46

[37] Friederich HC, Wu M, Simon JJ, Herzog W. Neurocircuit function in eating disorders. The International Journal of Eating Disorders. 2013;**46**(5):425-432

[38] Wierenga CE, Lavender JM, Hays CC. The potential of calibrated fMRI in the understanding of stress in eating disorders. Neurobiology of Stress. 2018;**9**:64-73

[39] Spalatro AV, Amianto F, Huang Z, D'Agata F, Bergui M, Abbate Daga G, et al. Neuronal variability of resting state activity in eating disorders: Increase and decoupling in ventral attention network and relation with clinical symptoms. European Psychiatry. 2018;**55**:10-17

[40] Peschel SK, Feeling NR, Vogele C, Kaess M, Thayer JF, Koenig J. A systematic review on heart rate variability in bulimia nervosa. Neuroscience and Biobehavioral Reviews. 2016;**63**:78-97

[41] Puviani L, Rama S, Vitetta GM. Computational psychiatry and psychometrics based on non-conscious stimuli input and pupil response output. Frontiers in Psychiatry. 2016;**7**:190

[42] Fonville L, Lao-Kaim NP, Giampietro V, Van den Eynde F, Davies H, Lounes N, et al. Evaluation of enhanced attention to local detail in anorexia nervosa using the embedded figures test; an FMRI study. PLoS One. 2013;**8**(5):e63964

[43] Warrier V, Grasby KL, Uzefovsky F, Toro R, Smith P, Chakrabarti B, et al. Genome-wide meta-analysis of cognitive empathy: Heritability, and correlates with sex, neuropsychiatric conditions and cognition. Molecular Psychiatry. 2018;**23**(6):1402-1409

[44] Rozenstein MH, Latzer Y, Stein D, Eviatar Z. Perception of emotion and bilateral advantage in women with eating disorders, their healthy sisters, and nonrelated healthy controls. Journal of Affective Disorders. 2011;**134**(1-3):386-395

[45] Dickson H, Brooks S, Uher R, Tchanturia K, Treasure J, Campbell IC. The inability to ignore: Distractibility in women with restricting anorexia nervosa. Psychological Medicine. 2008;**38**(12):1741-1748

[46] Bauer A, Schneider S, Waldorf M, Cordes M, Huber TJ, Braks K, et al. Visual processing of one's own body over the course of time: Evidence for the vigilance-avoidance theory in adolescents with anorexia nervosa? The International Journal of Eating Disorders. 2017;**50**(10):1205-1213

[47] Steward T, Menchon JM, Jimenez-Murcia S, Soriano-Mas C, Fernandez-Aranda F. Neural network alterations across eating disorders: A narrative review of fMRI studies. Current Neuropharmacology. 2018;**16**(8):1150-1163

[48] Renwick B, Campbell IC, Schmidt U. Review of attentional bias modification: A brain-directed treatment for eating disorders. European Eating Disorders Review. 2013;**21**(6):464-474

[49] Marucci S, Ragione LD, De Iaco G, Mococci T, Vicini M, Guastamacchia E, et al. Anorexia nervosa and comorbid psychopathology. Endocrine, Metabolic & Immune Disorders Drug Targets. 2018;**18**(4):316-324

Chapter 2

Bulimia Nervosa and Body Dissatisfaction in Terms of Self-Perception of Body Image

Layam Anitha, Asma Abdulaziz Alhussaini, Hessah Ibrahim Alsuwedan, Hessa Faleh Alnefaie, Rehab Abduallah Almubrek and Shima Abdulaziz Aldaweesh

Abstract

Bulimia nervosa is characterized by disturbed body image, repetitive binge eating, and compensatory behaviours such as self-induced vomiting, laxative abuse, or fasting. Body image dissatisfaction and eating disordered behaviours (e.g. food restriction, purging, and binge eating) can affect men and women of varied ages, races, and cultural backgrounds. Body dissatisfaction is defined as a negative subjective evaluation of the weight and shape of one's own body. Body dissatisfaction predicts the onset, severity, and treatment outcomes of eating disorders. A core component of body dissatisfaction is appearance-based social comparisons. In this context a study on self-perception of body image of women in Riyadh in 2018 revealed that a sudden spurt in obesity after marriage is leading to shift of higher percentage of women from positive to negative perception. Overall, an underestimation of body weight in terms of BMI was found among the participants. Such misconceptions should be addressed in view of the high obesity prevalence. It was also evident that positive and negative body image perception will lead to eating disorders in adolescents.

Keywords: self-perception, body image, misperception, BMI

1. Introduction

The diagnostic and statistical manual (DSM) [1] defines bulimia nervosa as characterised by disturbed body image, repetitive binge eating and compensatory behaviours such as laxative abuse, self-induced vomiting or fasting. Bulimia nervosa was ranked as 12th leading cause of disability adjusted life years (DALYs) in females aged 15–19 years in high income group countries out of 306 mental and physical disorders [2, 3]. Although this ranking did not change globally to a great extent between 1990 and 2013, ranking has been increased from 58th in 1990 to 46th in 2013 in low-income and middle income countries [2]. The review articles of eating disorders showed that it occurred mostly in the high-risk group of young western females [4, 5]. In 2014 Pike et al. found that eating disorders appear to be increasing in Asian and Arab countries in conjunction with increasing industrialization, urbanization and globalization [6]. In Europe, anorexia nervosa is reported by 1–4%, bulimia nervosa by 1–2% and Binge eating disorders (BED) by 1–4% of women [7]. The highest contributions of total DALY's caused by eating disorders among women aged 15–49 years was observed in India with over 1.32 billion, China over 1.38 billion along with United States [8]. Eating disorders have global distribution and are associated with increasing health burdens in Asia [9].

1.1 Association between bulimia nervosa, body image and body dissatisfaction

Body image has been studied extensively in patients with bulimia nervosa. Body image has been identified as an important factor in eating disorders but little research has been successfully carried out to have meaningful conclusions. Body image dissatisfaction and eating disordered behaviours can affect men and women of varied ages, races, and cultural backgrounds; however psychologists indicate that body image is one of the strongest gender differences in social sciences. Several studies have empirically investigated the role of social influence on body image and dissatisfaction [10]. Factors such as body-image dissatisfaction, the adoption of a perfectionistic attitude towards the body, the restrictive pursuit of thinness, and the development of bulimic tendencies are often indicated in scientific research as predictors of eating disorders [11–15]. However, most researchers focus on selected risk factors and indicate that the risk factors of eating disorders should not be considered separately. These factors seem to constitute the specific syndrome, related to the culture of thinness.

Body image is a multidimensional construct that represents body image evaluation that comprises perceptions, attitudes, and feelings about body size, shape and related behaviours [16]. The attitudinal dimension, also called as body satisfaction, reflects individuals' feeling about their body appearance, and the perceptual dimension is also called as body perception, which reflects individuals' subjective expectancy of their body image [17, 18]. Disturbances of body image perception are considered to be one of the central aspects of anorexia nervosa (AN) and bulimia nervosa (BN) [19]. According to Garner and Garfinkel [20], body image disturbances consist of two separate aspects, i.e. perceptual disturbance and body dissatisfaction. Perceptual disturbance involves the inability to assess the size of one's body accurately. Body dissatisfaction includes affective or attitudinal perceptions of one's body [20].

Body image disturbance (BID) refers to an overvaluation of one's appearance, possibly combined with difficulties in correctly gauging one's size and with pronounced body avoidance or checking behaviour. It is a transdiagnostic feature of AN and BN and assumed to be the core psychopathology of eating and weight disorders [21]. The distinction between body size distortion and body dissatisfaction has been studied in bulimic patients [12]. Although these two concepts have not been included in the DSM-III diagnostic criteria for bulimia nervosa, it has been postulated that a disturbance in body image plays a role in the disorder aetiology. Self-report procedures in the form of semi-structured interviews or questionnaires have been established for the assessment of BID, but experimental setups using specific devices are also commonly used [22, 23]. The different measures of BID are assumed to capture different aspects of BID.

Research has revealed associations between sociocultural aspects and women's perception towards body image. In some cultures, especially for women thinness is accepted as an icon of women whereas in other a medium body mass index (BMI) is accepted. It has been proposed that pressure to be thin from one's environment increases body dissatisfaction because the message to be thin via media or family fraternity will make the individual to feel discontent with their body image in terms of physical appearance. This view has been supported by perceived pressure leading to subsequent increase in body dissatisfaction [24] and in turn risk of development of an eating disorder [25]. A study was conducted by Massidda et al. [26] to analyse the relations between perceptual body distortion, body dissatisfaction, social influence and body Mass Index and the desire to change in a sample of young women. Results of this study revealed that participants tend to perceive their body as larger than real and they desire their body to be thinner than real which has been supported by Mikolajczyk et al. study [27]. Finally the results revealed that body dissatisfaction appears to be influenced both by social factors and BMI.

Previous research has reported both positive and negative aspects of body image as a psychological construct. A satisfactory body image has been linked to long term mental health and wellbeing [28, 29]. However body image dissatisfaction has been associated with a variety of disturbances that affect psychological functioning and quality of life which has led to unhealthy weight control behaviours and suicidal ideation [30, 31]. In general, people either have a positive or negative impression on the way they look. Some have learned how to be proud and tend to accept the way they look and feel about themselves regardless of what others might say or judge. On the other hand, people with a negative body image usually are dissatisfied. Thus, they tend to exaggerate the evaluation of their whole body or some parts whether bigger or smaller than what they actually are [32].

Based on the western study, women perceived themselves as '62% of overestimation' and '33% just right', while '5% of underestimation' compared with actual weight [33]. Furthermore, Saudi studies reported that only (23.3%) of the students had an agreement between their actual and perceived weight in which ideal body image discrepancies were found among the participants who wanted to be thinner (44.1%) or heavier (19.7%) than their perceived Body image [34]. Preference for a particular body weight and attitudes towards it may be mediated by cultural, personal and familial factors as well as an individual's own weight status [35].

Overall, the focus on ideal body size rather than on a range of acceptable body sizes has contributed to a literature that emphasizes female body size dissatisfactions [42]. Most of recent studies are conducted from western society. Since the issue of weight and weight perception are universal, the influence of social norms cannot be denied. Furthermore, there is a lack of information on how the misperception might affect Saudi women [43]. So, to understand self-perception, it is a demand to understand how people might feel about themselves as they definitely experience physical changes over their lifespan [46]. Study in south western in Saudi Arabia clarified that 76.7% had a disagreement in relation to misperception of body image [34]. Since it was highly significant in Saudi Arabia, where eating disorders and obesity is on increasing pace, it is incumbent to fill the gap and provide a reliable baseline data that might help the policy makers to develop an intervention program.

2. Methodology

A cross-sectional study was conducted in a university, located in Riyadh, Saudi Arabia. Participants are Saudi female from non-health college students and employees ranging in age from 18 to 50 years. The sample size was selected from open EPI website, based on confidence interval 95%. This study included 336 respondents out of which 269 (80%) were students and 67 (20%) were employees. Data was collected by structured self-administered questionnaire and close-ended questions. Some of the questions collected from previous studies and has been modified to be in line of Saudi culture. It includes socio-demographic information (ID, age, marital status, etc.), as well as, questions related to assessment of self-perception of body image, weight perception, socio-cultural factors affecting body image, lifestyle habits, body satisfaction and media influencers. The data was collected after receiving the approval from ethical committee of university.

3. Results and discussion

Results of the study are presented in terms of perceived and actual BMI (**Table 1**). According to actual measurement in students, the mean BMI was 23.72 = 8.63 (Mean = SD) which belong to normal and in employees, the mean was 27.27 + 5.69) which comes under the overweight category. The perceived mean BMI for students was 22.68 + 9.70, belong to normal and in employees, the mean was 25.74 + 6.05) which comes under the overweight category. The mean for BMI was less to students when compared to employees, though 47.8% of employees belong to 18–29 years of age. In the present study assessing body image self-perception BMI has been used as an indicator of nutritional status associated with determinants of body weight related behaviours. The mean actual BMI was more than the mean perceived BMI both in students and employees. When the perceived BMI is less than the actual and hence this can lead to increase in the obesity incidence in a long run. For preventing and reducing excess weight, the efficacy relies on one's realistic perception and self-awareness of their own body based on a real body size.

Body image was perceived as positive and negative in comparison with actual BMI of students. Out of 269 students, 71.6% have positive body image perception and 28.4% has negative body image perception. The difference between positive and negative body image perception was statistically significant at $x^2(3) = 43.37$, $p < 0.001$. Out of 66 employees, 56.1% have positive body image perception and 43.9% has negative body image perception and was statistically significant at $x^2(3) = 8.50$, $p = 0.03$. Percentage of positive perception towards body image was more when compared with negative perception in both the students and employees (**Figure 1**).

The question regarding the sociocultural view towards body image was asked as 'From 1 to 10 where you think the ideal BI rank according to your sociocultural perspective'. From the mentioned question 1–4 was represented as thin, 5–6 represented moderate and 7–10 as fat. According to actual BMI categories, 132 (40.6%) in normal weight responded that moderate weight is the ideal body in their society. Fat weight was the ideal body image responded by 27 (8.3%) participants of normal

Actual measurements	Students (N = 269)		Employees (N = 67)	
	M	SD	M	SD
Height	156.86	8.03	155.65	5.42
Weight	56.89	11.51	66.05	14.27
Waist circumference	71.89	8.86	82.06	12.14
BMI	23.42	8.63	27.27	5.69
Perceived measurements				
Height	158.7	8.77	157.52	7.23
Weight	56.07	11.01	63.79	14.87
BMI	22.68	9.7	25.74	6.05

Table 1.
Actual and perceived anthropometric measurements of students and employees.

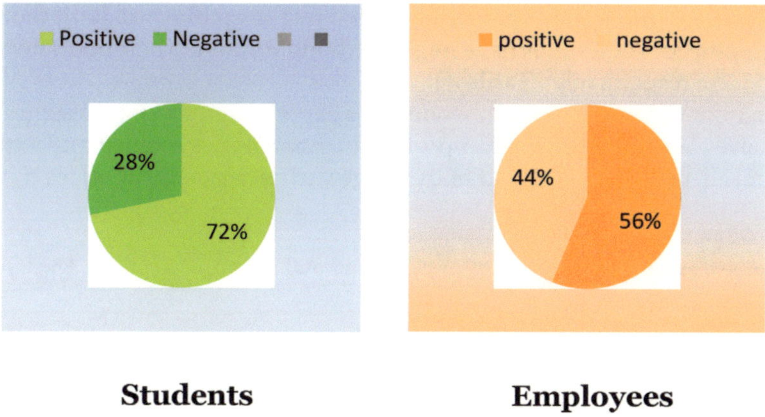

Figure 1.
Positive and negative perception towards body image among students and employees in PNU.

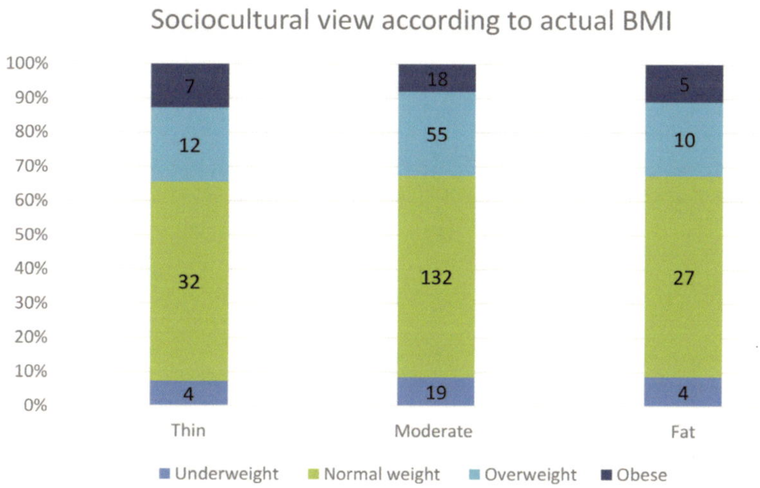

Figure 2.
Sociocultural view towards body image according to actual BMI categories among females.

weight category. Of normal weight category, thin weight was opted by 32 (9.9%) as ideal weight and only about 4 (1.2%) individuals from underweight category considered their weight as ideal weight (**Figure 2**). An interesting aspect observed from this study was 24.5% (55 in number) of overweight subjects rated that they belong to moderate scale of body image.

It is evident that 81% of students and 94% of employees felt that it appearance is very important, towards the perceptions of body image. Most of the percentage of the students that is 43.1–61.2% in employees wants to change their abdominal part and the good choice to change is through lose weight (48.7% in students and 68.7% in employees) (**Table 2**). 52% of students responded that media sometimes affect the perception of body image and 53.7% of employees responded the same. According to social pressure 49.8% of students responded that it never affects the body image. But 47.8% of employees responded that sometimes social pressure affects their body image (**Table 3**).

About 63.9% of students and 53.7% of employees responded that sometimes they compared their body shape with others. Lowered self-esteem is the highest (49.8%) consequence related to the negative perception of body image by students. Lowered self-esteem (37.3%) and gaining motivation to exercise, eat healthier, etc.

(35.8%) are the highest consequences reported by the employees. Both the students and the employees sometimes have negative thoughts about their bodies which is 59.9 and 58.2% respectively (**Table 4**).

Throughout the adult lifespan, women are experienced to various stages on how they perceive their body which is important to examine the implicit and explicit attitude of self-perception toward body image such as age, education level, marriage,

Importance of appearance	**Students**		**Employees**	
	N	**%**	**N**	**%**
Very important		81	63	94
Moderately important	45	16.7	3	4.5
Slightly important	5	1.9	0	0
Not important	1	0.4	0	0
Total	269	100	66	98.5
Body part wants to change				
Upper part	38	14.1	8	11.9
Abdominal part	116	43.1	41	61.2
Lower part	73	27.1	12	17.9
Nothing	40	14.9	5	7.5
Total	267	99.3	66	98.5
Prefer to				
Do nothing	21	7.8	2	3
Lose weight	131	48.7	46	68.7
Gain weight	40	14.9	4	6
Maintain as it is	77	28.6	14	20.9
Total	269	100	66	98.5

Table 2.
Descriptive statistics to assess the change towards their appearance of university students and employees.

Media affect	**Students**		**Employees**	
	N	**%**	**N**	**%**
Always	86	32	20	29.9
Sometimes	140	52	36	53.7
Never	42	15.6	10	14.9
Total	268	99.6	66	98.5
Social pressure				
Always	37	13.8	21	31.3
Sometimes	97	36.1	32	47.8
Never	134	49.8	13	19.4
Total	268	99.6	66	98.5

Table 3.
Descriptive statistics for social affect the body image perception of students and employees.

Comparing body shape with others	**Students**		**Employees**	
	N	%	N	%
Always	23	8.6	13	19.4
Sometimes	172	63.9	36	53.7
Never	73	27.1	17	25.4
Total	268	99.6	66	98.5
Consequences relate to negative perception of BI				
Being insecure around people	95	35.3	17	25.4
Embarrassment	37	13.8	9	13.4
General unhappiness	58	21.6	10	14.9
Lowered self –esteem	134	49.8	25	37.3
Undesirable to the opposite sex	13	4.8	2	3
Gaining motivation to exercise, eat healthier, etc.	94	34.9	24	35.8
How often do you think a negative thought about your body				
Always	18	6.7	13	19.4
Sometimes	161	59.9	39	58.2
Never	89	33.1	13	19.4
Total	268	99.6	66	97

Table 4.
Descriptive statistics indicate psychological effect of body image of students and employees.

pregnancy, social role changes, retirement, and menopause which can influence one's perceived level of body satisfaction [36, 37]. From social and psychological dimension, civilized and western societies are increasing the focus on female body image. They are inordinately emphasizing thinness as an ideal standard for beauty. Thus, women receive more social pressure to be beautiful than ever before [38, 39]. Regarding to social pressure, there was a study concerned about social factors and lifestyle associated with obesity among Arab women in Bahrain discovered that the ideal body is the middleweight, which found to be preferred more than thinness and fatness for women that are less socially accepted [34]. The revolution of mass media and fashion models has played an essential role on women perception towards their body image. The media is a powerful channel for transmission and reinforcement of cultural beliefs and values among all ages and ethnicities and other varieties, while it may not be exclusively responsible for determining the standards for physical attractiveness. Advertising, in particular creates a seductive and toxic mix of messages that can be taken seriously for both genders [40]. Nowadays, magazines, celebrities, idols all these agents contributes to make a difference in shaping our lives, changing beliefs and cultures in an imprescriptible way that we cannot even figure. Along with the ideal body image aspect which is being everywhere. A study investigated the satisfaction level in regard to BI among 10-year-old girls and boys. Unfortunately, they were dissatisfied with their bodies after watching their favourite actor or singer in a music video or clip from TV shows [41].

'Misperception of own weight status refers to the discordance between an individual's actual weight status and the perception of his/her weight status' [42]. The discoveries of misperception from a study conducted in Hail about body weight perception, among female university students has shown that, one-third of students misclassifying themselves when compared with actual weight [43]. Several studies show that female has a lot of curiosity about their body image and worried regarding it more than men. In 2014, a study conducted among Malaysian men and women found a misperception of own weight status and was higher among females (34.5%) compared to males (26.7%) [42]. According to the study, possible consequences might result in restrictive dieting and unhealthy weight control methods which may lead to increase the risk for the development of eating disorders, such as anorexia and bulimia nervosa [44]. Otherwise, underestimating one's own weight is associated with an increase of developing overweight prevalence [45]. Also, it is associated with depression, low self-esteem, feeling of shame, body surveillance, anxious and social isolation [40]. Additionally, Women's perception may shape into interpersonal relationship satisfaction [37].

4. Conclusions

Researchers believe that the body image of AN and BN individuals are characterised by distortion and disorder. BN is correlated largely with body image. In females due to high obesity percentages in some countries, characterized by more food intake, followed by depression, anxiety and hypochondriacally neurosis has led to body image distortion. Socio cultural factors largely contribute individual's perception in terms of body attractiveness which leads to more body self-image satisfaction or dissatisfaction. There is a statistically significant difference in students and employees towards their self-perception in terms of BMI and body image. Individuals with negative BI perception have functional correlations between the level of eating disorders and BI satisfaction.

Author details

Layam Anitha*, Asma Abdulaziz Alhussaini, Hessah Ibrahim Alsuwedan, Hessa Faleh Alnefaie, Rehab Abduallah Almubrek and Shima Abdulaziz Aldaweesh
Department of Health Sciences, College of Health and Rehabilitation Sciences, Princess Nourah University, Riyadh, KSA

*Address all correspondence to: layamanitha@gmail.com

References

[1] American Psychiatric Association. Diagnostic and Statistical Manual of Mental Disorders (DSM-5). 5th ed. Arlington, VA, USA: American Psychiatric Publishing; 2013

[2] Erskine HE, Whiteford HA, Pike KM. The global burden of eating disorders. Current Opinion in Psychiatry. 2016;**29**(6):346-353

[3] Murray CJL, Barber RM, Foreman KJ, et al. Global, regional, and national disability-adjusted life years (DALYs) for 306 diseases and injuries and healthy life expectancy (HALE) for 188 countries, 1990-2013: Quantifying the epidemiological transition. Lancet. 2015;**386**:2145-2191

[4] Smink FRE, Van Hoeken D, Hoek HW. Epidemiology, course and outcome of eating disorders. Current Opinion in Psychiatry. 2013;**26**:543-548

[5] Hoek HW. Epidemiology of eating disorders in persons other than the high risk group of young Western females. Current Opinion in Psychiatry. 2014;**27**:423-425

[6] Pike K, Hoek HW, Dunne PE. Recent cultural trends and eating disorders. Current Opinion in Psychiatry. 2014;**27**:436-442

[7] Keski-Rahkonen A, Mustelin L. Epidemiology of eating disorders in Europe: Prevalence, incidence, comorbidity, course, consequences and risk factors. Current Opinion in Psychiatry. 2016;**29**(6):340-345

[8] Thomas JJ, Lee S, Becker AE. Updates in the epidemiology of eating disorders in Asia and the Pacific. Current Opinion in Psychiatry. 2016;**29**(6):354-362

[9] Van Hoeken D, Burns JK, Hoek HW. Epidemiology of eating disorders in Africa. Current Opinion in Psychiatry. 2016;**29**(6):372-377

[10] Zydorczyk B, Sitnik-Warchulska K. Sociocultural appearance standards and risk factors for eating disorders in adolescents and women of various ages. Frontiers in Psychology. 2018;**9**:429. DOI: 10.3389/fpsyg.2018.00429

[11] Izydorczyk B. A psychological typology of females diagnosed with anorexia nervosa, bulimia nervosa or binge eating disorder. Health Psychology Report. 2015;**3**:312-325. DOI: 10.5114/hpr.2015.55169

[12] Stice E, Marti CN, Rohde P. Prevalence, incidence, and impairment a course of the proposed DSM-V eating disorder diagnoses in 8-year prospective community study of young women. Journal of Abnormal Psychology. 2013;**122**:445-457. DOI: 10.1037/a0030679

[13] Striegel-Moore RH, Roselli F, Perrin N, DeBar L, Wilson GT, Mag A, et al. Gender diferrence in the prevalaence of eating disorder symptoms. The International Journal of Eating Disorders. 2009;**42**:471-474. DOI: 10.1002/eat.20625

[14] Zechowski C. Polska wersja Kwestionariusza Zaburzenì od zywiania (EDI)–Adaptacja i normalizacja [polish version of eating disorder inventory–Adaptation and normalization]. Psychiatria Polska. 2008;**42**:179-193

[15] Jones DC, Crawford JK. The peer appearance culture during adolescence: Gender and body mass variations. Journal of Youth and Adolescence. 2006;**35**:257-269. DOI: 10.1007/s10964-005-9006-5

[16] Pruzinsky T, Cash TF. Understanding body images: Historical and contemporary perspectives. In: Cash TF, Pruzinsky T, editors. Body Image: A Handbook of Theory, Research, and Clinical Practice.

New York, NY: Guilford Press; 2002. pp. 3-12

[17] Ozmen D, Ozmen E, Ergin D, Cetinkaya AC, Sen N, Dundar PE, et al. The association of self-esteem, depression and body satisfaction with obesity among Turkish adolescents. BMC Public Health. 2007;7(80):1-7

[18] Gardner RM. Assessing body image disturbance in children and adolescents. In: Thompson JK, Smolak L, editors. Body Image, Eating Disorders, and Obesity in Children and Adolescents: Theory, Assessment, Treatment and Prevention. Washington D.C.: American Psychological Association; 2001. pp. 193-214

[19] Yamamotova A, Bulant J, Bocek V, Papezova H. Dissatisfaction with own body makes patients with eating disorders more sensitive to pain. Journal of Pain Research. 2017;**10**:1667-1675. DOI: 10.2147/JPR.S133425

[20] Garner DM, Garfinkel PE. Body image in anorexia nervosa: Measurement, theory and clinical implications. International Journal of Psychiatry in Medicine. 1981;**11**:263-284

[21] Fairburn CG, Cooper Z, Shafran R. Cognitive behaviour therapy for 640 eating disorders: A “trans diagnostic” theory and treatment. Behaviour Research and Therapy. 2003;**41**:509-528. DOI: 10.1016/s0005-6427967(02)00088-8

[22] Steinfeld B, Bauer A, Waldorf M, Hartmann AS, Vocks S. Diagnostik der Körperbildstörung. Psychotherapeut. 2017;**62**(3):164-182. DOI: 10.1007/s00278-017-0188-6

[23] Gaudio S, Brooks SJ, Riva G. Nonvisual multisensory impairment of 687 body perception in anorexia nervosa: A systematic review of 688 neuropsychological studies. PLoS ONE. 2014;**9**(10):e110087. DOI: 10.1371/journal.pone.0110087

[24] Stice E, Bearman SK. Body image and eating disturbances prospectively predict growth in depressive symptoms in adolescent girls: A growth curve analysis. Developmental Psychology. 2001;**37**:597-607

[25] Cash TF. Crucial considerations in the assessment of body image. In: Cash TF, Smolak L, editors. Body Image: A Handbook of Science, Practice, and Prevention. New York, NY: Guilford Press; 2011. pp. 129-137

[26] Massidda D, Bastianelli A, Vidotto G. Perceptual body distortion and body dissatisfaction: A study using adjustable partial image distortion. In: Conference: Fechner Day 2010 Department of General Psychology. Italy: University of Padova; 2010

[27] Mikolajczyk RT, Maxwell AE, Ansari WE, Stock C, Petkeviciene J, Guillen-Grima F. Relationship between perceived body weight and body mass index based on self-reported height and weight among university students: A cross-sectional study in seven European countries. BMC Public Health. 2010;**10**:40

[28] Mann MM, Hosman CM, Schaalma HP, De Vries NK. Self-esteem in a broad-spectrum approach for mental health promotion. Health Education Research. 2004;**19**(4):357-372

[29] Kirkcaldy BD, Shephard RJ, Siefen RG. The relationship between physical activity and self-image and problem behaviour among adolescents. Social Psychiatry and Psychiatric Epidemiology. 2002;**37**(11):544-550

[30] Cash TF, Morrow JA, Hrabosky JI, Perry AA. How has body image changed? A cross-sectional investigation of college women and men from 1983 to 2001. Journal of Consulting and Clinical Psychology. 2004;**72**(6):1081-1089

[31] Kim DS, Cho Y, Cho SI, Lim IS. Body weight perception, unhealthy weight control behaviors, and suicidal ideation

among Korean adolescents. The Journal of School Health. 2009;**79**(12):585-592

[32] Planned parenthood. Positive and Negative Body Image Improving Self Esteem. Planned parenthood, 2016. Available at: https://www.plannedparenthood.org/learn/body-image

[33] El-Ansari W, Clausen S, Mabhala A, Stock C. How do I look? Body image perceptions among university students from England and Denmark. International Journal of Environmental Research and Public Health. 2010;**7**(2):583-595

[34] Khalaf A, Westergren A, Berggren V, Ekblom O, Alhazzaa H. Perceived and ideal body image in among women in south western in Saudi Arabia. Journal of Obesity. 2015;**2015**:7. DOI: 10.1155/2015/697163

[35] Chang V, Christakis N. Self-perception of weight appropriateness in the United States. American Journal of Preventive Medicine. 2003;**24**(4):332-339

[36] Lee M. Women's body image throughout the adult life span: Latent growth modeling and qualitative approaches. Graduate Theses and Dissertations. 2013:13212. https://lib.dr.iastate.edu/etd/13212

[37] Howard T. Skin deep: Body image and interpersonal relationship quality in college women. Journal of Interdisciplinary Undergraduate Research. 2014;**6**(5):2

[38] Field A, Austin S, Camargo C, Tailor C, Striegel-Moore R, Loud K, et al. Exposure to the mass media, body shape concerns, and use of supplements to improve weight and shape among male and female adolescents. AAP News and Journals. 2005;**116**(2):e214-e220

[39] Wykes M, Gunter B. The Media and Body Image. Vol. 6. London: Sage Publications; 2005

[40] University of California Santa Crus. Student health outreach and promotion. University of California Santa Crus; 2015. Available from: http://shop.ucsc.edu/general-health-wellness/body-image.html.bodyimageimportant

[41] Long P, wall T. Media Studies, Texts, Production, Context, Producing Audiences: What Do Media Do to People? 2nd ed. London and New York: Routledge Taylor and Francis Group; 2012

[42] Shagar P, Shakiba N, Rahmah M. Factors associated with misperception of own weight status among 18-21 year old university students. IOSR Journal of Nursing and Health Science. 2014;**3**(5):25-31

[43] Epuru S, Eideh A, Shamsuddeen S, Al Shamarry S. Self-reported weight patterns and perceptions among female students of Saudi Arabia: A cross sectional survey. International Journal of Nutrition and Food Sciences. 2013;**2**(6):360

[44] Rand C, Resnick J. The "good enough" body size as judged by people of varying age and weight. Obesity Research. 2000;**8**(4):309-316

[45] Alwan H, Viswanathan B, Paccaud F, Bovet P. Is accurate perception of body image associated with appropriate weight-control behavior among adolescents of the Seychelles. Journal of Obesity. 2011;**2011**:8. DOI: 10.1155/2011/817242

[46] Slee P, Campbell M, Child SB. Adolescent and Family Development. 3rd ed. New York: Cambridge university press; 2012. p. 472

Chapter 3

Bulimia Nervosa: Is Body Dissatisfaction a Risk Factor?

Natalia Solano-Pinto, Miriam Valles-Casas and Raquel Fernández-Cézar

Abstract

Eating disorder studies are often carried out with adolescents. However, having a normal weight and the appearance of a seemingly healthy body makes many young people wait for years before seeking out professional consultation with a specialist. Therefore, after a review of the literature we will reflect on the role of body dissatisfaction in the development and persistence that occur in bulimia nervosa. It will be linked to the data found by our research group, both in samples of adolescents and adult women. Results on risk scores in purgative behaviors associated with bulimia nervosa, dieting, eating habits, physical activity, self-esteem, social skills, and body dissatisfaction will be described. They will be contrasted in a descriptive way with data from clinical study participants diagnosed with bulimia nervosa, leading to a predictive model of the role body dissatisfaction plays as a risk factor in the development of bulimia nervosa.

Keywords: body dissatisfaction, risk factor, predictive model, adolescents, adults

"After a lifetime of wanting to lose weight or 1 cm more around the waist, now I have other things to think about. My mind is out of jail and has many things to do".

"A woman fighting to overcome her illness."

1. Introduction

The first definition of the term "body image" is attributed to Schilder who defines it as follows: "the picture of our own body which we form in our own mind" ([1], p. 11). This author alludes to the mental representation of one's own body as a definition of body image. Currently, there is a general consensus that there is a multifactorial connotation attributed to this interpretation of body image in which cognitive, emotional, perceptive, and behavioral factors are interrelated [2]. Furthermore, the mental representation of the body is built on a basis of personal experience and the relationships with peer and adults, all of which are immersed in a specific sociocultural and historic context [3, 4]. In other words, the personal experience of one's own physical appearance is part of how we relate to others [5, 6].

The development of a positive body image is considered to be a public health issue by linking it to human well-being [7]. In fact, the existing research suggests that a negative development of body image constitutes a risk factor for psychological problems such as depression, suicidal thinking, low self-esteem, unhealthy behavior in order to control one's weight, and eating disorders [8]. Furthermore,

IntechOpen

body dissatisfaction is considered to be a predictor of physical inactivity and weight gain [9, 10]. It is also suggested that it is one of the most important factors for determining the persistence of eating disorders [11]. The prevalence of body dissatisfaction has been mainly studied in adolescence, considering people at this vital stage the main risk group for its development [12]. Thus, research places the prevalence among girls to be between 57 and 87% and among boys between 49 and 82% [13, 14]. However, in recent years, studies indicate an increase in the desire of boys to lose weight [15]. Along this line, [16] the silhouette scale was used with 1082 participants between 3 and 18 years of age and found that 61.2% presented dissatisfaction with their body with 44.7% of boys and 46% of girls expressing a desire to be thinner. Other research carried out with adults reported that body dissatisfaction is present in 60% of women and 40% of men [17].

The following will provide evidence to support the hypothesis that body dissatisfaction could be a risk factor for eating disorders, especially for bulimia nervosa.

2. Body dissatisfaction and associated factors

Over the past few years, researchers have focused their efforts on identifying the variables associated with the development of body dissatisfaction. Dion et al. [18] conducted a longitudinal study using an adapted version of the silhouettes scale with 413 participants between the ages of 14 and 18, obtaining the following results: one out of two girls wants to be thinner, and one in every five boys makes an attempt to lose weight. The factors that are mostly associated with body dissatisfaction in girls are: a desire to be thinner; the body mass index; exhibiting behaviors for losing weight; and negative comments about their weight. In the case of boys, some factors are: wanting to be thinner or bigger; the body mass index; having had sexual intercourse experiences; and negative comments about their own weight. Other authors, in an attempt to create predictive models in the development of body dissatisfaction, point out the effects that variables such as self-objectification, social comparison, internalization of what is considered to be "ideal beauty," and the perception that others have of the body and whether it will be accepted or rejected by them [19] have.

A key issue regarding body dissatisfaction is the standard of beauty. Previous studies have reported a positive correlation between the internalization of thinness ideal and the body dissatisfaction and symptoms of eating disorders, mainly in adolescents. In the work of Barajas-Iglesias et al. [21], carried out with a clinical sample of 104 patients aged 13–18 and diagnosed of anorexia nervosa (AN, n = 66) or bulimia nervosa (BN, n = 38), the authors claim that the influence of the esthetic body shape model is a relevant variable in eating disorders. In addition, they conclude that BN and AN patients are influenced by that model, but BN patients to a higher extent (94.74% BN vs. 68.18% AN). To sum up, the authors report that the esthetic body shape model relates to body dissatisfaction, and acts as a predictor of BN symptoms, especially purging behaviors (vomits, laxatives, or diuretics).

This canon of beauty is also associated with social, professional, and even personal success [20], and has the purpose of encouraging the consumption of esthetic treatments causing discrepancies between ideal beauty and the real body. As Vygotsky, the classic of evolutionary psychology indicates, the people, women and men as part of a given society, appropriate and internalize sociocultural norms making them their own, and normalize them as "appropriate" or expected [22]. In this vein, when a certain type of beauty is internalized, it becomes one's own ideal and becomes a need, rejecting other body forms that are far from that ideal.

In general, individuals immersed in a culture do not question the beauty guidelines offered in that culture; simply, and in a standardized way, the canon dictated by fashion is assumed.

This ideal-real body discrepancy is associated with body dissatisfaction in both, young people and adults [23]. In this sense, the internalization of an "ideal beauty" is accompanied by the rejection of any difference, being overweight or obese, and the mobilization of a plan to achieve a certain type of beauty. Aligned with that, a peculiar thinness is attributed to women, which is at odds with the biological and expected shapes of adult women: a sunken stomach, a disproportionately small waist in relation to the hips, large breasts in relation to the body's dimensions, etc. Also, in recent decades, men have exhibited their own contradictions in the attainment of the "ideal body" through a variety of means aimed at promoting muscle growth and thinness, with the most obvious discrepancies in having a full head of hair, muscular abs, and an absence of body hair [24]. In this line, people are educated to pay attention to their body shape, placing emphasis on what is supposedly deemed physically attractive, even if it means sacrificing functionality and competence. They are educated to consume and mold the body following a certain canon of beauty that is associated with success [25, 26].

These aspects, among others, are transmitted through media and technology, stories, toys, fashion, and the main educational and social agents: family, school, and peers [27, 28].

In the described context, social relationships are mediated by body image and awareness of weight [3]. Thus, when levels of dissatisfaction are high, the relationship with peers and the appreciation of friendship could be damaged by centering the conversation on the body, and making continuous comparisons between one's own body and that of others [14, 29]. In this respect, the person will relate addressing the desire to be liked, to be admired, with the fear of being rejected, and even with the risk of classifying and selecting friends based on body shapes [30]. In short, the individual internalizes that only through a certain body do they achieve success in their lives: have more friends, better jobs, more social or affective relationships. In addition, during childhood and adolescence, unfortunately, it is common to be the object of critical comments and ridicule toward the body, both in appearance and body competence. Having been the object of ridicule contributes to the development of body image based on dissatisfaction [31].

As previously mentioned, the family also contributes, explicitly or implicitly, to the development of body dissatisfaction: explicitly and directly, by comments and labels addressed to the body of their children, and implicitly, vicariously, or indirectly, through the treatment of their own body, as well as through dieting, doing exercise with the purpose of losing weight, flattery toward thin people, etc. [23, 32–34].

In the Critical Eye Research Group of Castilla La Mancha University, various researches in which the central theme has been body dissatisfaction have been carried out. In all the cases, the participants' informed consent has been obtained, under the principles of the Declaration of Helsinki. Fundamentally, the stages of life evaluated have been adolescence and adulthood. The project to assess body dissatisfaction in adults was performed with a non-probabilistic-intentional sample (233 adults, average age 32.4, 126 women and 107 men) composed by families from schools of Castilla La Mancha (España). The research has included the following instruments: a questionnaire to assess body dissatisfaction [35]; questions about having suffered teasing in childhood; items about muscle-building desire; and anthropometric measurements. Among the most relevant results are the following: 9.9% have marked or severe levels of body dissatisfaction. Compared to those with moderate levels, this group is characterized by being more overweight, having a greater desire for bodybuilding and a greater concern for physical appearance [36].

Along with that, 22.4% of the surveyed men report having been teased in their childhood, although this group is not characterized by high levels of dissatisfaction. In contrast, among women, 25.4% claim having suffered teasing, this group being characterized by high levels of dissatisfaction [37]. The results also indicate that in 22% of the families, at least one parent shows marked or severe levels of body dissatisfaction, a higher desire to be more muscular and a higher concern for health care [38].

Therefore, these results in adults indicate that body dissatisfaction is present in both men and women, and it has been noted that these data should be taken into account in health programs, as other research has also proposed. Similarly, the results obtained in adolescents indicate that body dissatisfaction should be a factor to consider in programs for the prevention of eating disorders and health promotion. This conclusion is reached by several authors. On the one hand, Valles and Solano-Pinto [39] who worked with a sample of 1040 young people, secondary education students from Castilla La Mancha (Spain) between the ages of 14 and 17 (55.7% women and 44.2% men), obtained results showing that 163 participants exhibited high levels of body dissatisfaction, out of which 110 were women and 53 were men, representing about 16% of the sample. On the other, Garner [40] worked with 406 participants with an average age of 12.2, early adolescence. Among this sample, 129 were men and 214 were women, evaluated with the EDI-2. In this case, 28 young people were considered as a group at risk of having severe levels of body dissatisfaction [41].

It seems, therefore, that the sociocultural pressure and the internalization of the desire to have a certain body type are so common that it is considered normal to feel dissatisfaction toward one's body, mainly in women, and increasingly in men. Such dissatisfaction, at moderate levels, is probably present because of the discrepancy between the proposed ideal body and the real one, for both men and women, in our society. The crucial aspect, in the context of eating disorders, is to detect the threshold: when the levels of body dissatisfaction are so high that one becomes obsessive and a possible risk factor for unhealthy behaviors and eating disorders such as bulimia nervosa [42]. If the desire for having a certain body is internalized in such a way that it becomes a necessity, the level of obsessiveness increases, the level of body dissatisfaction becomes so high that it could constitute a risk to one's health, triggering eating disorders.

3. Body dissatisfaction in bulimia nervosa

In light of this information, it seems that among the identified risks associated with body dissatisfaction is the development of eating disorders such as anorexia nervosa, bulimia nervosa, binge eating disorder, which primarily begin in adolescence, although they may also be present or triggered at other ages. In this sense, when the different components of body dissatisfaction in the adolescent population are evaluated through self-reporting [34], it has been shown that the probability of having an eating disorder is 32.2 times higher in young people with high scores in the behavioral component, compared to those with lower scores. For the perceptual component, the risk is 12.7 times higher, and for the cognitive-emotional component, the risk is 13.4 times higher [43].

Similar percentages are obtained in samples of adult women, for whom the risk of suffering the disorder increases by 22.5 when high scores are obtained from the IMAGE questionnaire. Additionally, 106 adult women were evaluated in the same study (55 diagnosed of eating disorders at a Spanish university hospital and 51 as a control group, estudiantes universitarias españolas), and it was observed that those diagnosed with bulimia nervosa obtained the highest scores in all the components of body dissatisfaction, that is, levels of body dissatisfaction in contrast to the diagnostic categories of anorexia nervosa, binge eating disorder or restrictive food intake disorder [44]. For this reason, some authors have emphasized the need to create differentiating profiles for each diagnostic category, considering high levels of internalization of sociocultural norms, social pressure toward the ideal body, and high levels of fear of maturity [21, 45, 46] as important factors for the onset of bulimia, along with body dissatisfaction. Parents' perception of their children's weight throughout childhood, concern about body weight and appearance in middle adolescence, and uncontrolled eating in late adolescence are also considered as predictive factors [47].

In the case of bulimia nervosa, in most people, the manifestations are activated with the decision to follow a strict diet that aims to modify the body quickly. According to some authors, such a decision would not occur if there were not a feeling of body dissatisfaction, that is, an experience of the body that implied discomfort and the desire to modify body forms [45, 46]. Thus, in general, the person varies their diet expecting a miraculous outcome, which will lead to a situation of imbalance, making the appearance of binge eating and vomiting likely. When there is a decrease in weight, and sometimes even without it, one receives a social compliment from the immediate environment that presumably interprets their weight loss or body change as an interest in taking care of their health. That compliment is seen as a reward for their efforts, a positive reinforcement, allowing for the persistence of the behavior to modify their body.

Occasionally, weight loss may have been accidental, due to a disease, or a situation that made it difficult to eat. But whether one starts from being overweight or from having a normal weight, social flattery occurs almost automatically. In addition, body dissatisfaction, which is at the heart of the decision, causes emotional malaise due to the anxiety that their body produces. As a result, in behavioral terms, a negative reinforcement is created when the anxiety is reduced through the modification of the body [48].

As already mentioned, all these situations are more critical in adolescence, which is considered a vital stage in the development of one's body image. This stage is characterized by strong biological, psychological, and social changes; identity is reaffirmed through the search for identification with a group that, in turn, identifies with role models, ways of spending their free time, ways of dressing, self-expression, etc., and in which the influence of the media and sociocultural aspects are of greater relevance. It is also the time when comments from their family and their peer group have the greatest impact on the person, because they are continually going back and forth between the need to be accepted, rule breaking, and group identification, all the while searching for their own individual identity. And in this search, teenagers have to choose how they want to be, what to believe in, who to relate to and how to relate to them, and whether they want to study and what they want to study. They are afraid, very afraid, of making mistakes, feeling rejected, or not feeling accepted. Sometimes, they do not build an identity, feeling out of control, or that they are incapable of facing life problems, and it is at these moments when the sociocultural influence overwhelms them and they can view the changes in their bodies, brought on by normal development, as undesirable. They selectively look at certain body areas as imperfect, compare their body shapes with those of their peers or social models, and feel insecure. They may resolve these conflicts provided that everything they have learned during childhood allows them to develop a protective shield, making them feel they have personal competence. This will depend, in part, on a positive development of body image in childhood. However, the feeling of insecurity or inferiority may also end up winning and make them feel that they are not good enough or worthy of being loved and accepted, and, as a result, this feeling of body inadequacy opens the door for unhealthy behaviors [31].

Therefore, some event that has made them feel especially bad about their body, or an occasional loss of weight (e.g. as a result of a mild illness such as the flu), may trigger the decision to diet or maintain weight loss, blaming their body for all their angst, and considering it to be the source of their problems. Now, with this new goal of modifying their body, they finally feel special; they feel that they are in control by building communication with and through the body and manipulating it. They turn this into their "project": a path to security and self-acceptance that they could not achieve through self-confirmation of their identity, even creating a sense of superiority over "all those people who don't have enough discipline to control themselves" [49].

The aspects commented so far on the role of body dissatisfaction in the development of bulimia nervosa are collected in **Figure 1**.

As indicated in **Figure 2**, thoughts and emotions about the body become progressively more repetitive, and negative beliefs about the body and weight are reactivated. It will become increasingly obsessive and generalized to different situations and in all areas of their life. That is, dissatisfaction with body image increases, and with it, the fear of gaining weight, which compels them to continue the diet. In this sense, the emotional angst caused by body dissatisfaction causes the person to develop an enormous fear of their body, which becomes predominant and augments the fear of gaining weight or of losing control [50].

As shown in **Figure 3**, as the disease takes hold, it is likely that there will be an excessive need for food, binge eating, real or perceived, which may be caused by an imbalance in the body as well as other factors. Such binge eating will initially be assessed as a situation of pleasure, of "forbidden taste" for food, which is also generally forbidden, and a negative reinforcement led by the reduction of the organic imbalance, of hunger [51]. However, after that, the binge eating is seen as

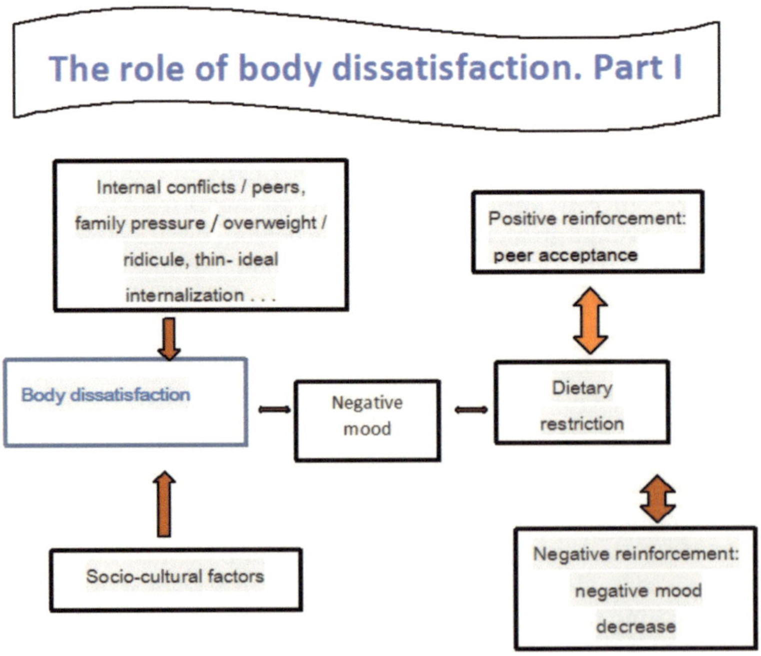

Figure 1.
The role of dissatisfaction. Part I.

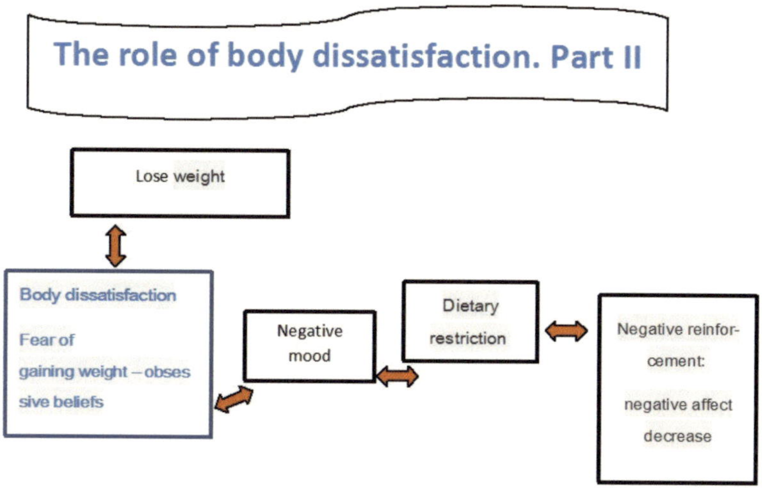

Figure 2.
The role of dissatisfaction. Part II.

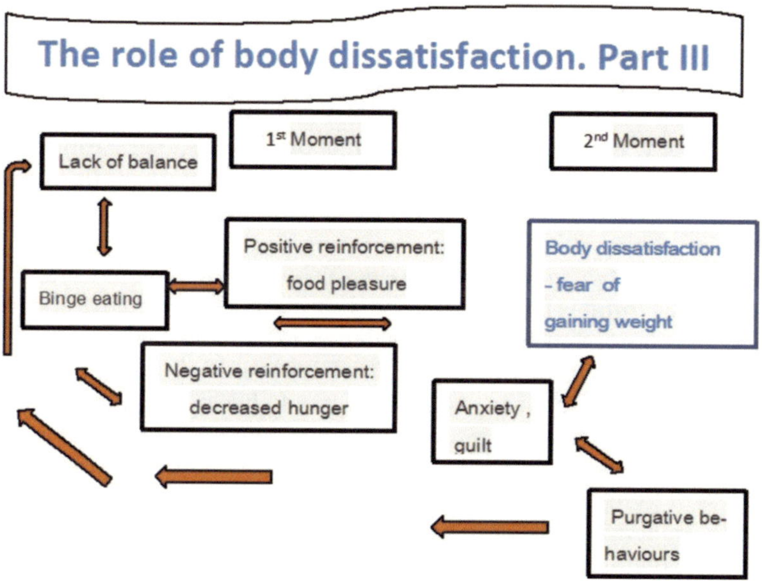

Figure 3.
The role of dissatisfaction. Part III.

an attack on the body: the obsessive beliefs about the body will be activated, and with them the emotional malaise. They are the insistent beliefs that one imposes on oneself regarding slimness, bodybuilding, and the rejection of obesity, all of which are greatly reinforced by current society and further compel the person to purge with the aim of reducing the anxiety and fear associated with weight gain [52].

The elements shown in **Figure 4** reflect that through the vicious circle of binge eating and purgative behaviors, one begins to formulate the erroneous belief that this is the only way that they can eat and not gain weight. Therefore, binge eating and purging will become more frequent and planned. Thoughts revolve around the need for having a certain body, and beliefs begin to emerge centering on the fact that eating a balanced diet will, irremediably, move them away from their goals. Given this, the role of stress must be considered. Whether caused or not caused

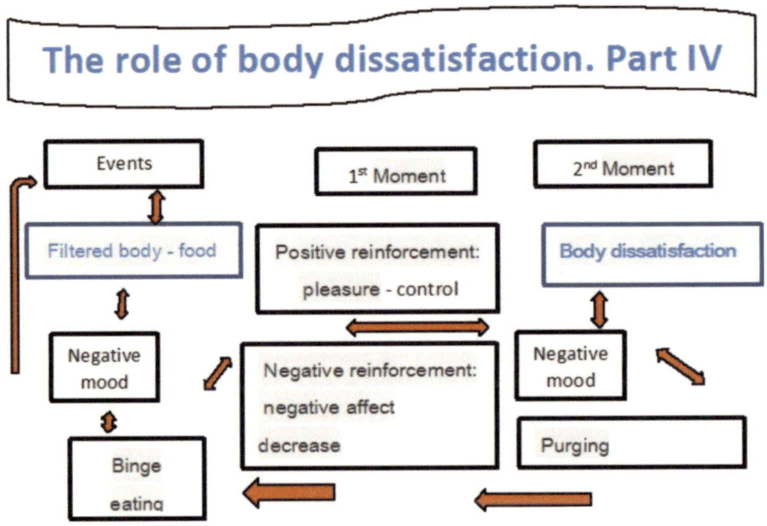

Figure 4.
The role of dissatisfaction. Part IV.

by the body, it is capable of generating anxiety that will increase the need to seek out other mechanisms for resolving the issue. Consequently, at different times, the problematic situation, whether or not it is related to the body, will be interpreted "through" the body. In this way, and depending on these interpretations, emotions of dissatisfaction, anxiety, sadness, and behaviors that sometimes become ritualistic will be awakened [53]. At the same time, emotions and behaviors reinforce distorted beliefs, being able to perceive suffering and pain as a source of pride, living in a dualism between mind and body: the body is undisciplined and must be controlled and the mind is fragmented in a dissociation between "a good me, and a bad me" [54]. In short, they live in ambivalence. What does the word ambivalence mean in this context? It is the internal debate between the desire to continue with one's objective of controlling the body, or to learn to live by accepting oneself.

In this ambivalence, family, friends, their boyfriends or girlfriends, teachers and professionals can accompany them by encouraging reflection on the suffering and loneliness of living through trying to control the body, and encouraging them to discover their identity, that they can be independent and live in their body in a healthy way. Following the interventions for improving body image which call for decreasing the internalization of sociocultural norms and social comparisons all the while learning to be unique (Stand-Alone), adolescents must be guided well by helping them to listen and interpret corporal sensations, accept their body shape and constitution, be critical of social pressure, confront comments that criticize the body or food, to block obsessive thoughts and to learn to look at themselves in a global way [55–57].

4. Conclusion

By living in a society, all people are exposed to sociocultural norms related to the body, aspects that influence and normalize a certain level of body dissatisfaction. As body dissatisfaction increases, it puts people at risk and moves them away from healthy behaviors. Fortunately, it only affects some people. There are those who will feel ill at ease with their body, but nothing else; others will learn to live with it; while others will intermittently follow restrictive diets. Only a small percentage will develop an eating disorder. Bulimia nervosa is, unquestionably, a disease with many factors that interact with one another and that, in a vital moment of vulnerability, increase the probability of developing the disease. In this chapter, a hypothetical model has been proposed that needs to be contrasted with future research. The role of body dissatisfaction in bulimia nervosa has been described, reflecting on the four phases of development of the disease, from the decision to lose weight to the use of binging and purging in an (unfortunate) attempt to self-regulate when facing everyday problems.

Given the results provided in the studies, it seems clear that body dissatisfaction can be considered a risk factor. It is also present once the disease has been developed, and it seems to maintain the typical manifestations of bulimia nervosa. But more research is needed, mainly longitudinal studies, to determine the role of different variables (anthropometric measurements, age, sex, anxiety, mood and personality traits, among others) in the development of body dissatisfaction. It is also necessary to know exactly what the relationship between body dissatisfaction and the manifestations of bulimia nervosa is in all phases of the disease, and if this dissatisfaction persists in people in clinical remission with respect to control groups. Such research should not be restricted to women, given the growing concern that men have been found to have with their own bodies.

Author details

Natalia Solano-Pinto[1], Miriam Valles-Casas[2] and Raquel Fernández-Cézar[1]*

1 Castilla La Mancha University, Faculty of Education, Toledo, Spain

2 Castilla La Mancha University, Faculty of Social Sciences, Talavera de la Reina, Spain

*Address all correspondence to: raquel.fcezar@uclm.es

References

[1] Schilder P. The Image and Appearance of the human body. Abingdon, OX (Oxon): Routledge; 1950/2000

[2] Wertheim EH, Paxton SJ. Body image development in adolescent girls. In: Cash TF, Pruzinsky T, editors. Body Image: A Handbook of Theory, Research, and Clinical Practice. New York, NY: The Guilford Press; 2011

[3] Raich RM. Imagen Corporal: Conocer y Valorar el Propio Cuerpo. Madrid: Pirámide; 2000

[4] Salazar Z. Adolescencia e imagen corporal en la época de la delgadez. Reflexiones. 2008;**87**:67-80

[5] Bulik C. The Woman in the Mirror. New York: Walker & Company; 2012

[6] Sidoli M. When the Body Speaks. London. Philadelphia: Routledge; 2000

[7] Molero D, Zagalaz-Sánchez ML, Cachón-Zagalaz JA. Comparative study of the physical self-concept across the life span. Revista de Psicología del Deporte. 2013;**22**(1):135-142

[8] Stice E, Marti CN, Durant S. Risk factors for onset of eating disorders: Evidence of multiple risk pathways from an 8-year prospective study. Behaviour Research and Therapy. 2011;**49**:622-627

[9] Grogan S. Body image and health: Contemporary perspectives. Journal of Health Psychology. 2006;**11**(4):523-530

[10] Van den Berg P, Neumark-Sztainer D. Fat on happy 5 years later: Is it bad for overweight girls to like their bodies? Journal of Adolescent Health. 2007;**41**(4):415-417

[11] Stice E, Whitenton K. Risk factors for body dissatisfaction in adolescent girls: A longitudinal investigation. Developmental Psychology. 2002;**38**:669-678

[12] Cash T. A negative body image: Evaluating epidemiological evidence. In: Cash T, Pruzinsky T, editors. Body Image: A Handbook of Theory, Research, and Clinical Practice. New York, London: The Guilford Press; 2002. pp. 269-276

[13] Almeida S, Severo M, Arau'jo J, Lopes C, Ramos E. Body image and depressive symptoms in 13-year-old adolescents. Journal of Paediatrics and Child Health. 2012;**48**:E165-E171

[14] Lawler M, Nixon E. Body dissatisfaction among adolescent boys and girls: The effects of body mass, peer appearance culture and internalization of appearance ideals. Journal of Youth and Adolescent. 2011;**40**:51-71

[15] Arrayás MJ, Tornero I, Díaz MS. Percepción de la imagen corporal de los adolescentes de Huelva atendiendo al género y a la edad. Retos. 2018;**34**:40-43

[16] López GL, Díaz A, Smith L. Análisis de imagen corporal y obesidad mediante las siluetas de Stunkard en niños y adolescentes españoles de 3 a 18 años. Anales de Psicología. 2018;**34**(1):167-172

[17] Tiggemann M. Body image across the adult life span: Stability and change. Body Image. 2004;**1**(1):29-41

[18] Dion J, Blackburn ME, Auclair J, Laberge L, Veillette S, Gaudreault M, et al. Development and etiology of body dissatisfaction in adolescent boys and girls. International Journal of Adolescence and Youth. 2015;**20**(2):151-166. DOI: 10.1080/02673843.2014.985320

[19] Andrew R, Tiggemann M, Clark L. Predicting body appreciation in young women: An integrated model of positive body image. Body Image. 2016;**18**:34-42

[20] Evans PC. "If only I were think like her, maybe I could be happy like her": The self-implications of associating a thin female ideal with life success. Psychology of Women Quarterly. 2003;**27**:209-214

[21] Barajas-Iglesias B, Jáuregui-Lobera I, Laporta-Herrero I, Santed-Germán MÁ. The influence of the aesthetic body shape model on adolescents with eating disorders. Nutrición Hospitalaria. 2018;**35**(5):1131-1137

[22] Da Silva R, Calvo S. La actividad infantil y el desarrollo emocional en la infancia. Revista Intercontinental de Psicología y Educación. 2014;**16**(2):19-30

[23] Lowes J, Tiggemann M. Body dissatisfaction, dieting awareness and the impact of parental influence in young children. British Journal of Health Psychology. 2003;**8**:135-147

[24] Silva DAS, Da Silva RC, Gonçalves ECA. Body image among men who practice body building: Comparison by age, economic statys and city size. Perceptual & Motor Skills: Perception. 2015;**121**(2):537-547

[25] O'Dea JA, Abraham S. Improving the body image, eating attitudes, and behaviors of young male and female adolescents: A new educational approach that focuses on self-esteem. International Journal of Eating Disorders. 2000;**28**(1):43-57

[26] Grogan S. Body Image. Understanding Body Dissatisfaction in Men, Women, and Children. London, New York: Routlege Psychology Press; 2008

[27] Jiménez-Moral JA, Zagalaz-Sánchez ML, Molero D, Pulido-Martos M, Ruiz JR. Capacidad aeróbica, felicidad y satisfacción con la vida en adolescentes españoles. Revista de psicología del deporte. 2013;**22**(2):429-436

[28] Mancilla-Medina A, Vázquez-Arévalo R, Mancilla-Díaz JM, Amaya-Hernández A, Alvarez Rayón G. Body dissatisfaction in children and preadolescents: A systematic review. Mexican Journal of Eating Disorders. 2012;**3**:62-79

[29] Chen LJ, Fox KR, Haase AM, Ku PW. Correlates of body dissatisfaction among Taiwanese adolescents. Asia Pacific Journal of Clinical Nutrition. 2010;**19**:172-179

[30] Jones DC. Interpersonal and familial influences on the development of body image. In: Cash TF, Smolak L, editors. Body Image. A Handbook of Science, Practice and Prevention. New York. London: The Guilford Press; 2011. pp. 110-119

[31] Toro J. El Adolescente Ante Su Cuerpo. Madrid: Pirámide; 2013

[32] Haines J, Neumark-Sztainer D, Hannan PJ, Robinson-O'Brien R. Child versus parent report of parental influences on children's weight-related attitudes and behaviors. Journal of Pediatric Psychology. 2008;**33**:783-788

[33] Smolak L. Body image development in childhood. In: Cash TF, Smolak L, editors. Body Image. A Handbook of Science, Practice and Prevention. New York, London: The Guilford Press; 2011. pp. 67-76

[34] Rodgers RF, Chabrol H. Parental attitudes, body image disturbance and disordered eating amongst adolescents and young adults: A review. European Eating Disorders Review. 2009;**17**:137-151

[35] Solano-Pinto N, Cano-Vindel A. IMAGEN. Evaluación de la insatisfacción con la imagen corporal. Madrid: TEA Ediciones; 2010

[36] Solano-Pinto N, Solbes-Canales I, Fernández-Cézar R, Calderón López

S, Pozo-Bardera C. Hábitos saludables en la primera infancia y en sus familias. Una invitación a la reflexión. DEMETRA. Food, Nutrition & Health. 2017;**12**(4):803-821. DOI: 10.12957/demetra.2017.28657

[37] Pozo C, Solano-Pinto N, Navarro C. Burlas in childhood and body dissatisfaction in adults. In: I International Congress of Intervention and Research in Health, 28 y 29 Septiembre 2017; Toledo. ISBN: 978-84-697-5272-2

[38] Solano-Pinto N, Solbes I, Calderón S, Fernández-Cézar R, Body dissatisfaction in families of children between 3 and 8 years. In: 3rd International Congress of Clinical and Health Psychology on children and adolescents; 16-18 Noviembre 2017; Sevilla. ISBN: 84-217-2848-5832

[39] Valles M, Solano-Pinto N (dir). Evaluación de actitudes y comportamientos asociados a los trastornos de conducta alimentaria. Memoria Para la obtencion de estudios avanzados. Albacete: Universidad de Castilla La Mancha; 2010

[40] Garner DM. Inventario de trastornos de la conducta alimentaria (EDI-2). Madrid: TEA Ediciones; 1998

[41] Valles M, Solano-Pinto N (dir). La imagen corporal: Proyecto preventivo sobre los trastornos de la conducta alimentaria [Tesis doctoral]. Albacete: Universidad de Castilla La Mancha; 2013

[42] Sepúlveda AR, Calado M. Westernization: The role of mass media on body image and eating disorders. In: Jáuregui-Lobera I, editor. Relevant Topics in Eating Disorders. InTech; 2012. pp. 47-64

[43] Solano-Pinto N, Cano-Vindel A, Blanco Vega H, Fernández Cézar R. Datos psicométricos de la versión abreviada del cuestionario IMAGEN; evaluación de la insatisfacción corporal. Nutrición Hospitalaria. 2017;**34**: 952-960. DOI: 10.20960/nh.695

[44] Solano-Pinto N, Cano-Vindel A, Bustamante E, Gómez del Barrio A. Evaluation of body dissatisfaction in the adult population with and without eating disorder with the IMAGEN questionnaire. In: Oral Communication Presented at IX Congreso Internacional de la Sociedad Española Para el Estudio de la Ansiedad y el Estrés; 6-8 Septiembre 2012; Valencia

[45] Izydorczyk B. A psychological profile of the bodily self-characteristics in women suffering from bulimia nervosa. In: Hay P, editor. New Insights into the Prevention and Treatment of Bulimia Nervosa. Croatia: InTech-Open Access Publisher; 2011. pp. 147-167

[46] Izydorczyk B. A psychological typology of females diagnosed with anorexia nervosa, bulimia nervosa or binge eating disorder. Health Psychology Report. 2015;**3**(4):312-325. DOI: 10.5114/hpr.2015.55169

[47] Allen KL, Byrne SM, Crosby RD. Distinguishing between risk factors for bulimia nervosa, binge eating disorder, and purging disorder. Journal of Youth and Adolescence. 2015;**44**:1580-1591. DOI: 10.1007/s10964-014-0186-8

[48] Stice E, Ng J, Shaw H. Risk factors and prodromal eating pathology. Journal of Child Psychology and Psychiatry. 2010;**51**:518-525

[49] Treasure J, Claudino AM, Zucker N. Eating disorders. Lancet. 2010;**375**:583-593

[50] Baker-Pitts. 'Look at me... What am I supposed to be?' Women, culture, and cosmetic plitting. In: Petrucelli J, editor. Body-States: Interpersonal/Relational Perspectives on the Treatment of Eating Disorders. London: Routledge; 2015. pp. 104-119

[51] Chernyak Y, Lowe MR. Motivations for dieting: Drive for thinness is different from drive for objective thinness. Journal of Abnormal Psychology. 2010;**119**:276-281

[52] Peñas-Lledó E, Aguera Z, Sánchez I, Gunnard K, Jiménez-Murcia S, Fernández-Aranda F. Differences in cognitive behavioral therapy dropout rates between bulimia nervosa subtypes based on drive for thinness and depression. Psychotherapy and Psychosomatics. 2013;**82**:125-126

[53] Stice E, Bohon C, Marti CN, Fischer K. Subtyping women with bulimia nervosa along dietary and negative affect dimensions: Further evidence of reliability and validity. Journal of Consulting and Clinical Psychology. 2008;**76**:1022-1033

[54] Hallings-Pott C, Waller G, Watson D, Scragg P. State dissociation in bulimic eating disorders: An experimental study. International Journal of Eating Disorders. 2005;**38**:37-41

[55] Alleva JM, Sheeran P, Webb TL, Martijn C, Miles E. A Meta-analytic review of Stand-Alone interventions to improve Body Image. PLoS ONE. 2015;**10**(9):e0139177. doi:10.1371/journal.pone.0139177

[56] Grabe S, Ward LM, Hyde JS. The role of the media in body image concerns among women: A metaanalysis of experimental and correlational studies. Psychol Bull. 2008;**134**(3):460-76. doi: 10.1037/0033-2909.134.3.460

[57] Irving LM, Berel SR. Comparison of media-literacy programs to strengthen college women's resistance to media images. Psychol Women Q, 2001;**25**(2):103-11

Section 2

The Neurobiology of Anorexia Nervosa: Insights into Pathophysiology and Novel Drug Targets

Chapter 4

The Neurobiology of Anorexia Nervosa

Ashley Higgins

Abstract

Anorexia nervosa is considered the most deadly psychological illness. Individuals with and recovered from anorexia nervosa experience numerous physical and mental health difficulties, and treatment outcomes remain unpromising. Anorexia nervosa is rare in the general population, but common among individuals with a first-degree relative with the disorder. In addition, the onset of anorexia nervosa is developmentally specific, which suggests a partly biological etiology. A better understanding of the biological and neurobiological etiology of anorexia nervosa is direly needed to inform new therapies and to identify individuals at risk for the disorder. This paper summarizes the research related to neurotransmitter abnormalities, aberrant brain activity, and genetic and epigenetic mechanisms that may contribute to the etiology of this deadly disorder.

Keywords: anorexia nervosa, neurobiology, neurotransmitters, genetics, etiology

1. Introduction

Anorexia nervosa (AN) is a serious psychological disorder characterized by low body weight, unhealthy weight loss methods, and an extreme focus on weight and body shape [1]. AN is associated with significant mortality risks due to medical complications, as well as the fact that one in five patients with AN die by suicide [2, 3]. The physical sequelae of AN, which are caused by self-starvation, affect nearly every major organ system. For instance, the gastrointestinal complications of AN include dysphagia [4], delayed gastric emptying [5], and risk of gastric dilation or even perforation [6]. Hematological and musculoskeletal complications include osteoporosis, fracture risk [7], and low red and white blood cell counts [8]. The endocrine system is impacted via elevated cortisol and growth hormones, low serum thyroid levels, and hypoglycemia [5, 9]. Dermatological complications include lanugo, acrocyanosis, and thinning hair [10]. Neurological complications, which will be discussed in depth throughout this chapter, are well-documented in terms of the effects of long-terms caloric restriction on brain volume and neural activity [11]. Finally, cardiac complications, which are most often linked to mortality in AN, include bradycardia [12], prolonged QTc interval [13], and left ventricular atrophy [14].

Current medication and psychotherapies have limited success in treating AN. The prognosis is especially poor if treatment begins more than 3 years after the onset of symptoms [15]. AN currently has no viable treatment options [16], as current medications and psychotherapies provide only minor to modest effects, with especially poor outcomes among women with entrenched AN [16–18]. It is estimated that only half of individuals with AN achieve full remission of symptoms, and even recovered patients typically maintain a low weight and experience chronic depressive symptoms [19]. Given the lack of viable treatment options for AN, leading eating disorders researchers are now recommending that future research focus on identification of risk factors and other preventive strategies [20, 21].

Many of the identified risk factors for AN are biological or genetic in nature. AN is a rare disorder, with estimated lifetime prevalence ranging from 0.1 to 3.6%, and a point prevalence rate ranging from 0.1 to 1.2% in the general population [22]. Though the overall prevalence of AN is quite low, AN represents the third most common chronic illness with adolescent onset [23]. In addition, the risk of AN is elevated among individuals with a family history of AN. It is a well-documented finding that AN tends to run in families [24, 25]. Some studies have found a 10-fold risk of AN among first-degree relatives of individuals with the disorder [26–28] or an overall heritability of 0.56 [25]. Furthermore, AN has a developmentally specific age of onset. Taken together, these findings suggest the presence of biological and/or genetic risk factors in the etiology of AN [29].

Individuals with AN often display a relentless pursuit of further weight loss and believe themselves to be overweight even when they are emaciated. In addition to pathological eating patterns, individuals with EDs also experience a host of unusual symptoms, such as "(1) extremes of behavioral inhibition and dysinhibition; (2) anxiety, depression, and obsessionality; and (3) puzzling symptoms such as body image distortion, perfectionism, and anhedonia" ([30], p. 38) as well as "intense body-focused anxiety, self-disgust, compulsive behavior and altered information processing—i.e. raised pain threshold, reduced sense of taste, anosognosia, inability to integrate thoughts and feelings, poor visuospatial memory, cognitive rigidity and weak central coherence" ([31], p. 580). Any biological mechanisms accounting for the inherent eating pathology of AN should also modulate these emotional and cognitive phenomena.

Identifying true risk factors for AN presents a complicated methodological problem. By definition, a risk factor must be present prior to the onset of illness, and identifying these factors prior to the symptom onset requires a prospective design [32]. However, given the low prevalence rate of AN, prospective studies are often too complicated to perform; thus, the research literature on AN risk factors is often limited to retrospective studies, with their inherent bias in retrospective recall [33].

Another methodological approach samples from individuals who have recovered from AN (RECAN). While recovery from AN is a long and ill-defined process, more than half of individuals with AN are able to completely or partly achieve remission [34]. Individuals RECAN are assumed to no longer be experiencing the sequelae of the starvation state. However, the use of individuals RECAN is limited as a methodological approach in that "scar" effects from a period of illness could be misidentified as premorbid risk factors [35]. In order to circumvent the possibility of "scar" effects, studies must identify endophenotypes that are present among individuals with active AN, individuals RECAN, and among unaffected family members [36, 37]. Utilizing this approach, several potential endophenotypes have been identified, by eliminating any neurobiological findings that improve with refeeding and identifying abnormalities that are shared by individuals with AN and their unaffected family members [16].

Many of the neurobiological phenomena to be discussed in this paper are present premorbidly, exaggerated by malnutrition, and return to premorbid levels after recovery [38]. There are currently promising lines of research on dopaminergic [29], serotonergic [39], and noradrenergic pathways [31], as well as dysregulations in appetitive functioning [30], genetic and epigenetic contributions [40, 41], contributions from gonadal hormones [42], and aberrations in brain activity [43].

2. Dopamine

Dopaminergic functioning modulates reward and affect, and an aberration in dopaminergic functioning has been implicated in obsessive or ritualistic behaviors, such as the food rituals observed in individuals with AN [29]. It seems intuitive that reward functioning is impaired in AN, as individuals with AN often present as abstemious, anhedonic, and temperate in a multitude of behaviors even in childhood, long before the onset of symptoms [44]. Dopamine is central in processing reward in both primary and secondary reinforcers, including food [45–47]. Several research studies have revealed altered striatal dopamine function in individuals with and RECAN [29, 48, 49]. Ingestion of highly palatable foods, such as high-sugar foods, may trigger dopamine release in individuals without AN; this release of dopamine in response to food is similar to the release of dopamine elicited by amphetamine use, which is often associated with feelings of euphoria [50]. However, among individuals RECAN, amphetamine use triggers the expected endogenous dopamine release, but this release of dopamine is experienced as highly unpleasant and anxiogenic [51]. If similar processes take effect during exposure to highly palatable food, which would be experienced as highly anxiogenic to individuals with AN, this could partially account for the persistence that individuals with AN display in their pursuit of self-starvation; if food is anxiogenic, self-starvation downregulates this anxiety. Whereas individuals without AN experience pleasure from foods, individuals with AN find it aversive. Thus, the reinforcing aspects of food are not experienced by individuals with active AN or individuals RECAN.

Reward processing in general appears to be altered in individuals with AN, even in situations that do not involve food- or weight-related cues. In fMRI research, individuals RECAN failed to differentiate between winning and losing money in a gambling task [52]. Therefore, individuals with AN may have a diminished ability to identify the positive or negative value of a stimulus. Individuals with AN fail to show appropriate appetitive motivational system activation to a variety of cues [49]. Thus, altered dopaminergic function reflects high conditioning of reward for disease-salient stimuli, but a failure to respond appropriately to other positive and negative cues [18].

Among individuals RECAN, dopamine metabolite concentrations in the cerebral spinal fluid remain depleted years after the disorder [53]. Perhaps to correct for this depletion, dopamine 2 and 3 (D_2/D_3) receptor binding in the ventral striatum is elevated among individuals RECAN [44]. At this time there are no publications on dopamine aberrations in unaffected family members. However, animal models of anorexia strongly suggest a dopaminergic endophenotype, as administering dopamine antagonists in activity-based anorexia in rats facilitates increased food intake [54]. This hints at a dopaminergic role in promoting weight loss, which can be reversed with psychopharmacology that acts on the dopamine system.

3. Serotonin

Additionally, serotonergic (5-HT) dysfunction may be a biological marker for AN. Serotonin has seemed a likely candidate for some time, given this neurotransmitter's active influence in modulating mood and appetite [29]. A recent meta-analysis has concluded that being a carrier of the S allele of the 5-HTTLPR polymorphism of the serotonin transporter gene is predictive of eating disorders, particularly anorexia [55]. The gene coding of the serotonin transporter (5-HTT) works in the presynaptic neuron to terminate serotonin activity in the synapse and recycle serotonin back into the presynaptic neuron. 5-HTT is coded by a gene on chromosome 17, and the 5-HTTLPR polymorphism of this gene has the greatest impact on behavior. The S allele is a short variant of this 5-HTTLPR polymorphism, which decreases the availability of 5-HTT and results in dysphoria.

In terms of appetite, any treatment that increases intrasynaptic 5-HT or activates 5-HT receptors will reduce appetite and food consumption, while any treatment that reduces transmission or blocks receptors will promote weight gain [56]. Caloric restriction has an enormous impact on the available serotonin in the brain [29]. Tryptophan is one of 20 essential amino acids and can be absorbed only through caloric intake, especially carbohydrate intake [57]. Tryptophan, through a series of chemical processes, becomes serotonin. A restricted diet limits the amount of tryptophan (and, therefore, the amount of serotonin) that is available to the brain [58]. In addition, a restricted diet decreases the rate of synthesis in serotonin receptors and the density of serotonin transporters, which results in oversensitivity to serotonin in postsynaptic receptors [59]. Not surprisingly, individuals in the acutely ill state have lowered concentrations of the 5-HT metabolite 5-HIAA in the cerebral spinal fluid [56]. However, elevated levels of 5-HIAA were likely present premorbidly. Individuals with AN premorbidly report high levels of anxiety, dysphoria, and obsessionality, which are associated with high levels of 5-HT in the synapse [42]. Dieting actually serves to regulate the 5-HT in the synapse. This reduction of serotonin, in the short term, results in anxiolytic effects for people who restrict calories [29]. These anxiolytic effects could explain why individuals with AN cling so desperately to their restrictive behaviors: these behaviors are inadvertently medicating underlying anxiety.

The serotonin system includes at least 14 different receptors. The 5-HT_{1A} and 5-HT_{2A} receptors appear most influential in the pathogenesis of AN. The 5-HT_{1A} autoreceptor serves to decrease 5-HT transmission [56]. Individuals with AN have 50–70% more binding at these receptors, and retain 20–40% more binding after recovery. In addition, the 5-HT_{1A} receptor may play a role in the efficacy of selective serotonin reuptake inhibitors (SSRIs), which are potently effective at treating depression and anxiety [60, 61]. While starvation decreases 5-HT across the brain, the overactive 5-HT_{1A} receptor continues to inhibit 5-HT transmission. The combination of these forces is so powerful that SSRIs exert minimal impact in increasing intrasynaptic 5-HT, which fails to provide symptom relief for individuals with AN [56]. In AN, SSRIs fail to desensitize 5-HT_{1A} receptors, which inhibits presynaptic 5-HT.

Newer imaging technologies, such as PET imaging with selective neurotransmitter radioligands, allow for viewing in vivo neurotransmitter activity in the brain. Postsynaptic 5-HT_{2A} receptors have been studied in this way. The 5-HT_{2A} receptor has been afforded special attention because activity at this receptor is influential in two of the central, yet most perplexing, symptoms of AN: poor problem-solving abilities and distorted body image [62, 63]. 5-HT_{2A} receptor binding is reduced in several brain areas, especially in the cingulate and temporal regions. The cingulate-temporal dysfunction could be related to inefficient problem-solving behaviors among individuals with AN, who struggle with incorporating affective and social stimuli into tasks [64]. Individuals with AN do not seem to learn from mistakes, but stubbornly and obsessively use the same strategies, despite poor results. This could indicate dysfunction in executive functioning and planning. In terms of distorted body image, which is characterological for individuals with AN, 5-HT_{2A} disturbances in the left parietal region of the brain are thought to be responsible [62]. Lesions in the right parietal region have been associated with neglect, which could be theoretically related to body image distortion, especially if this information is coded in the parietal regions of each hemisphere [56]. The activity at 5-HT_{2A} receptors remains dysregulated even after a year of maintaining normal weight, regular menstruation, and no binge/purging/restricting. Prolonged dysregulation at these receptors may partially account for the inefficacy of SSRIs in treating AN, regardless of the phase of the disorder [17, 18].

Additionally, serotonergic dysfunction is common to other psychiatric concerns, especially those that are likely to be comorbid with AN, such as major depression [65] and anxiety disorders [66]. While abnormalities in serotonergic functioning are common to all of these disorders, different patterns of serotonergic functioning emerge on a molecular level [67]. While 5-HT_{1A} receptor binding is often decreased in individuals with or recovered from depression [68, 69] and panic disorder [70], 5-HT_{1A} receptor binding is increased in individuals with AN [29]. This could indicate that serotonergic dysfunction is a common vulnerability for a variety of disorders, with disorder-specific patterns at the neuronal level. This also accounts for higher rates of psychiatric concerns among family members of individuals with AN.

Given etiological research on the separate roles of dopamine and serotonin, it is not surprising that the most recent research suggests that interactions between serotonin and dopamine activity truly elicit and maintain the eating pathology of AN [56]. This interaction is not well understood, but could hold promise for future pharmacological interventions for AN.

4. Norepinephrine

Based on previous research on dopaminergic and serotonergic dysfunction in individuals with active AN, individuals RECAN, and unaffected family members, it is safe to conclude that neurotransmitter activity is aberrant both during the premorbid, active, and recovery periods of AN. Dopaminergic and serotonergic pathways could account for some, though not all, of the core symptoms of AN [29, 42]. While these pathways (particularly the serotonergic pathway) partly account for rigidity and perfectionism among individuals with AN, individuals with AN display a variety of perplexing symptoms that seem unrelated to both the starvation state itself or serotonin dysfunction alone; individuals with AN report difficulty with pain perceptual, alexithymia, reduced sense of taste, as well as numerous other perplexing symptoms [31]. Aberrant activity in the noradrenergic pathway could better account for this vast range of deficits.

Norepinephrine is a neurotransmitter which serves multiple functions in the body and brain, including regulation of sympathetic arousal/anxiety and cerebral blood flow [71]. Norepinephrine levels are elevated premorbidly in AN [72], but appear to be decreased in plasma and cerebrospinal fluid during active AN ad RECAN [72–74]. Premorbidly high levels of norepinephrine lead to high sympathetic arousal and anxiety [31]. Among individuals with AN, this anxiety is often focused on food- and weight-related issues, though the inherently high trait levels of perfectionism and neuroticism can manifest in other achievement domains such as schoolwork or sports [75]. Since this anxiety is linked an abundance of norepinephrine, dieting in the early stages of AN counteracts this by depleting the brain of the precursors to norepinephrine that are normally ingested through food [31]. Dieting is then maintained through negative reinforcement, leading to a reduction in body weight and entrenchment of AN symptoms. Furthermore, aberrant activity in the noradrenergic system has been linked to irregular patterns of activation in the insula, which will be discussed in the next section.

5. Brain volume, blood flow, and neural activity

Various neuroimaging studies show substantial structural abnormalities in the brain among individuals with active AN [30, 76, 77]. However, significant questions remain as to:

> *whether such anomalies reflect regionally specific disturbances that might help explain disorder-defining psychopathology or merely generic, global consequences of malnutrition. Similarly, it remains unclear whether structural alterations in AN constitute premorbid traits or persisting "scars," as might be the case if they would still be evident following weight restoration ([76], p. 214).*

Decreased volumes of white and gray brain matter have been documented throughout the brain during the acute phases of illness [77, 78]. More specifically, gray matter atrophy has been noted in the cerebellum, hypothalamus, caudate nucleus and frontal, parietal and temporal areas [77, 79, 80], as well as in the cingulate cortex [81] and the precuneus [82]. The rate of gray matter atrophy is not uniform across the brain during active AN; atrophy in the hypothalamus may appear early in AN, whereas atrophy in the cerebellum is a late consequence of AN among patients with longer durations of illness [77].

However, these gray and white matter findings appear to be specific to the acute phase of illness and caused by malnutrition and cerebral dehydration [77]. A meta-analysis revealed that gray matter is reduced by 5.6% during the acute phases of AN, whereas white matter is reduced by 3.8% [83]. A few months of treatment and results in approximately 50% of gray matter regain and nearly all of the white matter being regained. A few years following remission of AN, gray matter and white matter depletions are no longer statistically significant. It is possible that hormone levels impact how much gray matter is recovered, as high levels of cortisol at the time of hospitalization are negatively correlated with gray matter restoration following weight gain [84]. All told, the decreased volume of white and gray matter in individuals with AN normalizes with proper nutrition [38, 85]. Thus, these gray and white matter findings are not likely to be a contributing factor to the neurobiological etiology of AN.

In contrast, abnormal patterns of blood flow to the brain and brain activity persist after recovery. For instance, individuals who have recovered from AN often have hypoperfusion in the frontal, parietal, temporal and occipital areas of the brain [86]. In addition, overactivation of the frontal and anterior cingulate cortex (ACC) and insula following exposure to pictures of food or the taste of food is present both during active AN and after recovery [87, 88]. Hyperactivity in these regions could be an endophenotype for AN and be related to more global difficulties with appetitive mechanisms.

The complex eating pathology inherent in AN may indicate atypical functioning in appetitive mechanisms. Despite the unique and stereotypic presentation of altered eating patterns in the eating disorder diagnoses, it is still unknown whether individuals with AN have disordered appetitive functioning. The neural and limbic circuits are more likely candidates for deregulating appetitive functioning in AN than peripheral signs (such as hormonal imbalances or abnormalities in the gastrointestinal tract), because these neural and limbic circuits also regulate reward processing and emotionality, which are known to be disordered in AN [89]. Individuals with AN display an almost phobic avoidance of high-fat foods, which persists after recovery. Individuals who have recovered from AN fail to connect hunger cues with positive ratings of food [88]. Particularly promising research has focused specifically on the anterior insula, which is positioned in the primary gustatory cortex [90]. While this is still debated, researchers posit that the anterior insula codes a representation of food and its hedonic value, and projects to other parts of the brain [91, 92]. The anterior insula resides next to the orbito-frontal cortex, which interprets information from the anterior insula and is responsible for flexible decision-making with ever-changing stimuli [93]. Put another way, the anterior insula represents the food and its hedonic value, while the orbito-frontal cortex weighs those representation against hunger and other variables. Critically, the orbito-frontal cortex is very sensitive to changes in serotonin, which could account for the inflexibility in eating pathology in individuals with AN [94]. Even though research in this area is still in its infancy, the aforementioned processing abnormalities in the anterior insula and orbito-frontal cortex shed some light as to how "AN individuals fail to become appropriately hungry when starved, and thus are able to become emaciated" ([30], p. 45).

Though disturbances related to the gustatory modulation of the anterior insula certainly appear to be a key part of a biological risk factor in AN, the anterior insula influences many processes unrelated to gustatory mechanisms [30]. Disturbances in the anterior insula could be related to a more general deficit in interoceptive awareness [95, 96]. Altered activity in the insula "supports the idea that they might suffer from a fundamentally and physiologically altered sense of self" ([97], p. 111). Some of the more mysterious symptoms of AN, such as a denial of signs of malnutrition and lack of motivation to change pathological eating behaviors, could be linked to abnormal patterns of activity in the insula [98].

6. Genetics

There is clear and compelling evidence that having a first-degree relative with AN significantly elevates one's risk for developing AN; in fact, relatives of individuals with AN are 11.3 times more likely to develop AN [27]. There is likely some genetic contribution to the etiology of AN. Current heritability estimates range between 50 and 80% [99, 100], though specific genetic mechanisms have been difficult to identify. A noteworthy paradox was pointed out regarding the high heritability of AN and the likelihood of reduced reproductive fitness from prolonged periods of malnutrition [101]. Thus, one can conclude that genes that contribute to the etiology of AN must be rare and of recent origin. In addition, high rates of diagnostic crossover between eating disorder categories (see [102]) and high rates of comorbidity with mood and anxiety disorders (see [103]) also complicate the genetic etiology of AN, since any genetic predispositions for AN should be non-specific and shared with these other conditions.

One method of identifying genes relevant to the pathophysiology of AN is the candidate gene approach. The candidate gene approach is defined as an examination of genes that could be involved in a particular disease or syndrome because the function of those genes is related to the sequelae of the illness [104]. The candidate gene approach could be likened to finding "a needle in the haystack" of 27,000 human genes. Thus, it is not surprising that candidate gene studies for AN are controversial and many fail to replicate genetic association.

Family-based linkage analyses, or the process of detecting the location of disease genes on the chromosome, have identified three chromosomal regions of interest for AN; one resides on chromosome 13 (specifically, 13q13.3) and is related to drive-for-thinness, another resides on chromosome 2 (2p11.2) and is related to obsessionality, and a third on chromosome 1 (specifically, 1q1.3) which is related to both obsessionality and drive-for-thinness [105].

Genes related to dopamine transfer (DAT1) and dopamine receptors (DRD2) have been examined among patients with AN. Individuals with AN show elevated expression of DAT1 and reduced expression of DRD2 [106]; while the implications of these expression are not fully understood, a genetic contribution to the etiology of AN related to dopamine expression is consistent with previously mentioned research on altered reward processing in AN. Other genetic research has also identified an interaction of three genes that clear serotonin and norepinephrine from the synapse; these genes (a serotonin transporter gene, a norepinephrine transporter gene, and a monoamine oxidase A gene) appear to contribute to the risk of restricting AN [41]. While the presence of each gene variant alone is associated with a somewhat increased risk of restricting AN, the combination of all three gene variants leads to a risk that is up to eight times greater than the risk associated with one gene variant alone.

Finally, there are epigenetic factors to consider. Perhaps the most important epigenetic mechanism to consider is the role of estradiol in triggering genetic risk for AN, which is discussed below. All told, the genetic and epigenetic contributions to AN remain largely unknown. Genetic studies are limited by previously mentioned methodological issues, such as the low prevalence of AN and the near impossibility of recruiting individuals with AN during the premorbid period for genetic research. However, progress in identifying genes or patterns of gene expression could lead to pharmacological advances that are direly needed for this population given the poor response to common psychotropics such as selective serotonin reuptake inhibitors, tricyclic antidepressants, and antipsychotics [17, 18].

7. Pubertal hormones

The vast majority of individuals with AN are biologically female and begin experiencing symptoms of AN during the pubertal and pre-pubertal periods of development [1]. These findings suggest that gonadal hormones specific to females may play a role in the epigenesis of AN. It is possible that genetic factors may be more impactful for females than males with regards to drive for thinness and body dissatisfaction [107] as well as for concerns about body shape and weight [108]. In addition to gender differences in genetic factors, genetic risk for eating disorders appears to be moderated by age, as there is almost no genetic effect (5% or less on disordered eating among preadolescent female twins, but by late adolescence there is evidence of substantial genetic effects [109]. Upon closer examination, the genetic effect appears to be due to pubertal status and not age, as 11-year-old twins who had begun puberty showed a higher magnitude of genetic effects compared to same-age twins who had not begun puberty [110]. Pubertal hormones, such as estradiol, which steadily increases during puberty among females, may trigger the genetic risk for disordered eating, as high levels of estradiol are associated with magnitude of genetic effects in a manner independent of age and physical signs of puberty development, such as body hair or breast development [111].

In addition to triggering the genetic risk for AN, low estradiol levels are associated with a number of negative effects during the active phases of AN. Not surprisingly, malnourished individuals show a variety of hormonal imbalances, most of which return to baseline after recovery [42]. Pubertal hormones appear to follow this same pattern of alteration during active illness but return to baseline upon weight regain. In a typically developing adolescent, an increase in pubertal hormones aids in brain maturation, most notably in the limbic system [112, 113]. These hormone levels are altered among individuals diagnosed with AN, who may experience amenorrhea due to low body weight and/or body fat [114]. When individuals achieve weight regain and recommence with menstruation, cognitive functioning improves, suggesting that increasing levels of estradiol during weight regain may assist with neural recovery [115].

8. Conclusions and future directions

The etiology of AN is multifaceted, with contributions from genetic factors, biological factors, family dynamics, personality characteristics, and sociocultural influences. The development of this disorder and its maintenance remain poorly understood despite a significant increase in rigorous scientific study into risk factors and shared vulnerabilities with other eating disorders and psychological disorders.

In recent years, the neurobiological etiology of AN has been examined through a wide variety of imaging studies, genetic studies, and hormonal/biological studies (see [97]). A number of key findings are summarized in this paper. Across these studies, it is clear that the brains of individuals with AN show evidence of altered reward processing and appetitive mechanisms, which are linked to a number of dopaminergic findings (perhaps, most importantly, how the brains of individuals with AN process cues of palatable foods as highly anxiogenic and aversive [50, 51]. Serotonergic functioning has been long-thought to account for behavioral rigidity and trait obsessionality in AN [56], and recent genetic research has identified a number of potential serotonergic genetic candidates or interactions of genetic candidates that represent significant risk factors for AN [44, 74, 104, 107]. Finally, altered noradrenergic functioning and aberrant activity in the insula represent a unique but comprehensive view of the global difficulties individuals with AN have with emotions, insight, and interoceptive awareness [31, 71]. These findings, taken together, can illuminate future pathways for pharmacotherapies that will be more effective for individuals with AN. Other brain-based findings discussed in this paper, such as gray and white matter atrophy, are unlikely to represent true risk factors, because the vast majority improve with proper nutrition.

In conclusion, the neurobiological etiology of AN in-and-of-itself is complex and complicated by factors such as the low prevalence rate of AN [1], lack of prospective research [32], and the at-times catastrophic impact of malnutrition on the brain and body [38]. AN continues to be considered the most deadly psychological illness, and individuals RECAN may face a lifetime of physical and emotional challenges [1]. Given the ego-syntonic nature of this disorder and that current treatment outcomes are suboptimal for this population, a better understanding of the biological vulnerabilities of this illness and the development of new therapies are direly needed.

Conflict of interest

There are no conflicts of interest to report.

Author details

Ashley Higgins
Immaculata University, Malvern, PA, United States of America

*Address all correspondence to: ahiggins@immaculata.edu

References

[1] American Psychiatric Association. Diagnostic and Statistical Manual of Mental Disorders. 5th ed. Washington, DC: American Psychiatric Association; 2013

[2] Arcelus J, Mitchell AJ, Wales J, Nielsen S. Mortality rates in patients with anorexia nervosa and other eating disorders: A meta-analysis of 36 studies. Archives of General Psychiatry. 2011;**68**:724-731. DOI: 10.1001/archgenpsychiatry.2011.74

[3] Franko DL, Keshaviah A, Eddy KT, Krishna M, Davis MC, Keel PK, et al. A longitudinal investigation of mortality in anorexia nervosa and bulimia nervosa. American Journal of Psychiatry. 2013;**170**:917-925. DOI: 10.1176/appi.ajp.2013.12070868

[4] Holmes SR, Gudridge TA, Gaudiani JL, Mehler PS. Dysphagia in severe anorexia nervosa: A case report. International Journal of Eating Disorders. 2012;**45**:463-466. DOI: 10.1002/eat.20971

[5] Westmoreland P, Krantz MJ, Mehler PS. Medical complications of anorexia nervosa and bulimia. The American Journal of Medicine. 2016;**129**:30-37. DOI: 10.1016/j.amjmed.2015.06.031

[6] Mascolo M, Dee E, Townsend R, Brinton JT, Mehler PS. Severe gastric dilatation due to superior mesenteric artery syndrome in anorexia nervosa. International Journal of Eating Disorders. 2015;**48**:532-534. DOI: 10.1002/eat.22385

[7] Faje AT, Fazeli PK, Miller KK, Katzman DK, Ebrahimi S, Lee H, et al. Fracture risk and areal bone mineral density in adolescent females with anorexia nervosa. International Journal of Eating Disorders. 2014;**47**:458-466. DOI: 10.1002/eat.22248

[8] Hutter G, Ganepola S, Hofmann WK. The hematology of anorexia nervosa. International Journal of Eating Disorders. 2009;**42**:293-300. DOI: 10.1002/eat.20610

[9] Lo Sauro C, Ravaldi C, Cabras PL, Faravelli C, Ricca V. Stress, hypothalamicpituitary-adrenal axis and eating disorders. Neuropsychobiology. 2008;**57**:95-100. DOI: 10.1159/000138912

[10] Strumia R. Eating Disorders and the Skin. New York, NY: Springer; 2012

[11] Fuglset TS, Endestad T, Hilland E, Bang L, Tamnes CK, Landrø NI, et al. Brain volumes and regional cortical thickness in young females with anorexia nervosa. BMC Psychiatry. 2016;**16**:404-412. DOI: 10.1186/s12888-016-1126-9

[12] Yahalom M, Spitz M, Sandler L, Heno N, Roguin N, Turgeman Y. The significance of bradycardia in anorexia nervosa. The International Journal of Angiology. 2013;**22**:83-94. DOI: 10.1055/s-0033-1334138

[13] Krantz MJ, Sabel AL, Sagar U, Long CS, Barbey JT, White KV, et al. Factors influencing QT prolongation in patients hospitalized with severe anorexia nervosa. General Hospital Psychiatry. 2012;**34**:173-177. DOI: 10.1016/j.genhosppsych.2011.08.003

[14] Lamzabi I, Syed S, Reddy VB, Jain R, Harbhajanka A, Arunkumar P. Myocardial changes in a patient with anorexia nervosa: A case report and review of literature. American Journal of Clinical Pathology. 2015;**143**:734-737. DOI: 10.1309/AJCP4PLFF1TTKENT

[15] Treasure J, Russell G. The case for early intervention in anorexia nervosa: Theoretical explanation of maintaining factors. British Journal of Psychiatry.

2011;**199**:5-7. DOI: 10.1192/bjp.bp.110.087585

[16] Bulik C, Berkman ND, Brownley KA, Sedway JA, Lohr KN. Anorexia nervosa treatment: A systematic review of randomized control trials. International Journal of Eating Disorders. 2007;**40**:310-320. DOI: 10.1002/eat

[17] Holtkamp K, Konrad K, Kaiser N, Ploenes Y, Heussen N, Grzella I, et al. A retrospective study of SSRI treatment in adolescent anorexia nervosa: Insufficient evidence for efficacy. Journal of Psychiatric Research. 2005;**39**:303-310. DOI: 10.1016/j.jpsychires.2004.08.001

[18] Kaye WH, Frank GK, Bailer UF, Henry SE. Neurobiology of anorexia nervosa: Clinical implications of alternations of the function of serotonin and other neuronal systems. International Journal of Eating Disorders. 2005;**37**:S15-S19. DOI: 10.1002/eat.20109

[19] Novotney A. New solutions: Psychologists are developing promising new treatments and conducting novel research to combat eating disorders. Monitor on Psychology. 2009;**40**:46. Available from: http://www.apa.org/monitor/2009/04/treatments.aspx

[20] DeSocio JE, O'Toole JK, Nemirow SJ, Lukack ME, Magee MJ. Screening for childhood eating disorders in primary care. Primary Care Companion to the Journal of Clinical Psychiatry. 2007;**9**:16-20. DOI: 10.4088/PCC.v09n0103

[21] Fleming M, Towey K, editors. Educational Forum on Adolescent Health: Adolescent Obesity, Nutrition, and Physical Activity. Chicago, IL: American Medical Association; 2003

[22] Dahlgren CL, Wisting L, Rø Ø. Feeding and eating disorders in the DSM-5 era: A systematic review of prevalence rates in non-clinical male and female samples. Journal of Eating Disorders. 2017;**5**:56-65. DOI: 10.1186/s40337-017-0186-7

[23] Nicholls D, Viner R. ABC of adolescence: Eating disorders and weight problems. British Medical Journal. 2005;**330**:950-953. DOI: 10.1136/bmj.330.7497.950

[24] Bulik CM, Sullivan PF, Wade TD, Kendler KS. Twin studies of eating disorders: A review. International Journal of Eating Disorders. 2000;**27**:1-20. DOI: 10.1002/(SICI)1098-108X(200001)27:1<1::AID-EAT1>3.3.CO;2-H

[25] Bulik C, Sullivan PF, Tozzi F, Furberg H, Lichtenstein P, Pedersen NL. Prevalence, heritability, and prospective risk factors for anorexia nervosa. Archives of General Psychiatry. 2006;**63**:305-312. DOI: 10.1001/archpsyc.63.3.305

[26] Lilenfeld LR, Kaye WH, Greeno CG, Merikangas KP, Plotnicov K, Pollice C, et al. A controlled family study of anorexia nervosa and bulimia nervosa: Psychiatric disorders in first-degree relatives and effects of proband comorbidity. Archives of General Psychiatry. 1998;**55**:603-610. DOI: 10.1001/archpsyc.55.7.603

[27] Strober M, Freeman R, Lampert C, Diamond J, Kaye W. Controlled family study of anorexia and bulimia nervosa: Evidence of shared liability and transmission of partial syndromes. American Journal of Psychiatry. 2000;**157**:393-401. DOI: 10.1176/appi.ajp.157.3.393

[28] Strober M, Freeman R, Lampert C, Diamond J, Kaye W. Males with anorexia nervosa: A controlled study of eating disorders in first-degree relatives. International Journal of Eating Disorders. 2001;**29**:263-269. DOI: 10.1002/eat.1017

[29] Kaye WH. Neurobiology of anorexia and bulimia nervosa. Physiology and Behavior. 2008;**94**:121-135. DOI: 10.1016/j.physbeh.2007.11.037

[30] Kaye W, Wagner A, Fudge JL, Paulus M. Neurocircuitry of eating disorders. In: Adan RA, Kaye WH, editors. Behavioral Neurobiology of Eating Disorders. New York, NY: Springer; 2011. pp. 37-57

[31] Nunn K, Frampton I, Lask B. Anorexia nervosa—A noradrenergic dysregulation hypothesis. Medical Hypotheses. 2012;**78**:580-584. DOI: 10.1016/j.mehy.2012.01.033

[32] Jacobi C, Hayward C, de Zwaan M, Kraemer HC, Agras WS. Coming to terms with risk factors for eating disorders: Application of risk terminology and suggestions for a general taxonomy. Psychological Bulletin. 2004;**130**:19-65. DOI: 10.1037/0033-2909.130.1.19

[33] Anderluh MB, Tchanturia K, Rabe-Hesketh S, Collier D, Treasure J. Lifetime course of eating disorders: Design and validity testing of a new strategy to define the eating disorders phenotype. Psychological Medicine. 2009;**39**:105-114. DOI: 10.1017/S0033291708003292

[34] Franko DL, Tabri N, Keshaviah A, Murray HB, Herzog DB, Thomas JJ, et al. Predictors of long-term recovery in anorexia nervosa and bulimia nervosa: Data from a 22-year longitudinal study. Journal of Psychiatric Research. 2018;**96**:183-188. DOI: 10.1016/j.jpsychires.2017.10.008

[35] Kaye WH, Greeno CG, Moss H, Fernstrom J, Fernstrom M, Lilenfeld LR, et al. Alterations in serotonin activity and psychiatric symptoms after recovery from bulimia nervosa. Archives of General Psychiatry. 1998;**55**:927-935. DOI: 10.1001/archpsyc.55.10.927

[36] Lilenfield LR. Personality and temperament. In: Adan RA, Kaye WH, editors. Behavioral Neurobiology of Eating Disorders. New York, NY: Springer; 2011. pp. 3-16

[37] Lilenfeld LR, Stein D, Bulik CM, Strober M, Plotnicov K, Pollice C, et al. Personality traits among currently eating disordered, recovered and never ill first-degree female relatives of bulimic and control women. Psychological Medicine. 2000;**30**:1399-1410. DOI: 10.1017/S0033291799002792

[38] Wagner A, Greer P, Bailer UF, Frank GK, Henry SE, Putnam K, et al. Normal brain tissue volumes after long-term recovery in anorexia and bulimia nervosa. Biological Psychiatry. 2006;**59**:291-293. DOI: 10.1016/j.biopsych.2005.06.014

[39] Grice DE, Halmi KA, Fichter MM, Strober M, Woodside DB, Treasure JT, et al. Evidence for a susceptibility gene for anorexia nervosa on chromosome 1. American Journal of Human Genetics. 2002;**70**:787-792. DOI: 10.1086/339250

[40] Tenconi E, Santonastaso P, Monaco F, Favaro A. Obstetric complications and eating disorders: A replication study. International Journal of Eating Disorders. 2015;**48**:424-430. DOI: 10.1002/eat.22304

[41] Urwin R, Nunn K. Epistatic interaction between the monoamine oxidase A and serotonin transporter genes in anorexia nervosa. European Journal of Human Genetics. 2005;**13**:370-375. DOI: 10.1038/sj.ejhg.5201328

[42] Kaye W, Fudge J, Paulus M. New insights into symptoms and neurocircuit function of anorexia nervosa. Nature Reviews Neuroscience. 2009;**10**:573-584. DOI: 10.1038/nrn2682

[43] Nunn K, Frampton I, Fugslet T, Torzsok-Sonnevand M, Lask B. The

insula hypothesis of anorexia nervosa. Medical Hypotheses. 2011;**76**:353-357. DOI: 10.1016/j.mehy.2010.10.038

[44] Frank G, Bailer UF, Henry S, Drevets W, Meltzer CC, Price JC, et al. Increased dopamine D2/D3 receptor binding after recovery from anorexia nervosa measured by positron emission tomography and [^{11}C]ralopride. Biological Psychiatry. 2005;**58**:908-912. DOI: 10.1016/j.biopsych.2005.05.003

[45] Schultz W. Neural coding of basic reward terms of animal learning theory, game theory, microeconomics, and behavioural ecology. Current Opinion in Neurobiology. 2004;**14**:139-147. DOI: 10.1016/j.conb.2004.03.017

[46] McClure S, Berns G, Montague P. Temporal prediction errors in a passive learning task activate human striatum. Neuron. 2003;**38**:339-346. DOI: 10.1016/S0896-6273(03)00154-5

[47] O'Doherty J. Reward representations and reward-related learning in the human brain: Insights from neuroimaging. Current Opinion in Neurobiology. 2004;**14**:769-776. DOI: 10.1016/j.conb.2004.10.016

[48] Bergen A, Yeager M, Welch R, Haque K, Ganjej JK, Mazzanti C, et al. Association of multiple DRD2-141 polymorphisms with anorexia nervosa. Neuropsychopharmacology. 2005;**30**:1703-1710. DOI: 10.1038/sj.npp.1300719

[49] Friederich HC, Kumari V, Uher R, Riga M, Schmidt U, Campbell IC, et al. Differential motivational responses to food and pleasurable cues in anorexia and bulimia nervosa: A startle reflex paradigm. Psychological Medicine. 2006;**36**:1327-1335. DOI: 10.1017/S0033291706008129

[50] Avena NM, Bocarsly ME. Dysregulation of brain reward systems in eating disorders: Neurochemical information from animal models of binge eating, bulimia nervosa, and anorexia nervosa. Neuropharmacology. 2012;**63**:87-96. DOI: 10.1016/j.neuropharm.2011.11.010

[51] Bailer UF, Narendran R, Frankle WG, Himes ML, Duvvuri V, Mathis CA, et al. Amphetamine induced dopamine release increases anxiety in individuals recovered from anorexia nervosa. International Journal of Eating Disorders. 2012;**45**:263-271. DOI: 10.1002/eat.2093

[52] Wagner A, Aizenstein H, Venkatraman M, Fudge J, May J, Mazurkewicz L, et al. Altered reward processing in women recovered from anorexia nervosa. American Journal of Psychiatry. 2007;**164**:1842-1849. DOI: 10.1176/appi.ajp.2007.07040575

[53] Kaye WH, Frank GK, McConaha C. Altered dopamine activity after recovery from restricting-type anorexia nervosa. Neuropsychopharmacology. 1999;**21**:503-506. DOI: 10.1016/S0893-133X(99)00053-6

[54] Verhagen LA, Luijendijk MC, Hillebrand JJ, Adan RA. Dopamine antagonism inhibits anorectic behavior in an animal model for anorexia nervosa. European Neupsychopharmacology. 2009;**19**:153-160. DOI: 10.1016/j.euroneuro.2008.09.005

[55] Calati R, De Ronchi D, Bellini M, Serretti A. The 5-HTTLPR polymorphism and eating disorders: A meta-analysis. International Journal of Eating Disorders. 2011;**44**:191-199. DOI: 10.1002/eat.20811

[56] Bailer UF, Kaye WH. Serotonin: Imaging findings in eating disorders. Current Topics in Behavioral Neurosciences. 2011;**6**:59-79. DOI: 10.1007/7854_2010_78

[57] Markus CM. Dietary amino acids and brain serotonin function:

Implications for stress-related affective changes. Neuromolecular Medicine. 2008;**10**:247-258. DOI: 10.1007/s12017-008-8039-9

[58] Kiezebrink K, Mann ET, Bujac SR, Stubbins MJ, Campbell DA, Blundell JE. Evidence of complex involvement of serotonergic genes with restrictive and binge/purge subtypes of anorexia nervosa. World Journal of Biological Psychiatry. 2010;**11**:824-833. DOI: 10.3109/15622975.2010.484550

[59] Haleem DJ. Exaggerated feedback control decreases brain serotonin concentration and elicits hyperactivity in a rat model of diet-restriction-induced anorexia nervosa. Appetite. 2008;**52**:44-50. DOI: 10.1016/j.appet.2008.07.009

[60] Cipriani A, Furukawa TA, Salanti G, Geddes JR, Higgins JP, Churchill R, et al. Comparative efficacy and acceptability of 12 new-generation antidepressants: A multiple-treatments meta-analysis. The Lancet. 2010;**373**:746-758. DOI: 10.1016/S0140-6736(09)60046-5

[61] Cuijpers P, Straten A, Warmerdam EH, Andersson G. Psychological treatment versus combined treatment of depression: A meta-analysis. Depression & Anxiety. 2009;**26**:279-288. Available from: http://dspace.ubvu.vu.nl/handle/1871/16593

[62] Bailer UF, Price JC, Meltzer CC, Mathis CA, Frank GK, Weissfeld L, et al. Altered 5-HT_{2A} receptor binding after recovery from bulimia-type anorexia nervosa: Relationships to harm avoidance and drive for thinness. Neuropsychopharmacology. 2004;**29**:1143-1155. DOI: 10.1038/sj.npp.1300430

[63] Frank G, Kaye WH, Meltzer CC, Price JC, Greer P, McConaha C, et al. Reduced 5-HT_{2A} receptor binding after recovery from anorexia nervosa. Biological Psychiatry. 2002;**52**:896-906. DOI: 10.1016/S0006-3223(02)01378

[64] Klump KL, Bulik CM, Pollice C, Halmi KA, Fichter MM, Berrettini WH, et al. Temperament and character in women with anorexia nervosa. Journal of Nervous and Mental Disorders. 2000;**188**:559-567. DOI: 10.1097/00005053-200009000-00001

[65] Tremblay LK, Naranjo CA, Graham SJ, Hermann N, Mayberg HS, Hevenor SJ, et al. Functional neuroanatomical substrates of altered reward processing in major depressive disorder revealed by a dopaminergic probe. Archives of General Psychiatry. 2005;**62**:1228-1236. DOI: 10.1001/archpsyc.62.11.1228

[66] Stein M, Simmons A, Feinsteim J, Paulus M. Increased amygdala and insula activation during emotion processing in anxiety-prone subjects. American Journal of Psychiatry. 2007;**164**:318-327. DOI: 10.1176/appi.ajp.164.2.318

[67] Phillips M, Drevets WR, Lane R. Neurobiology of emotion perception I: The neural basis of normal emotion perception. Biological Psychiatry. 2003;**54**:504-514. DOI: 10.1016/S0006-3223(03)00168-9

[68] Sargent PA, Kjaer KH, Bench CJ, Rabiner EA, Messa C, Meyer J, et al. Brain serotonin$_{1A}$ receptor binding measure by positron emission tomography with [^{11}C]WAY-100635: Effects of depression and antidepressant treatment. Archives of General Psychiatry. 2000;**57**:174-180. DOI: 10.1001/archpsyc.57.2.174

[69] Bhagwagar Z, Rabiner E, Sargent P, Grasby P, Cowen P. Persistent reduction in brain serotonin 1_A receptor binding in recovered depressed men measured by positron emission tomography with [^{11}C]WAY-100635. Molecular Psychiatry. 2004;**9**:386-392. DOI: 10.1038/sj.mp.4001401

[70] Neumeister A, Brain E, Nugent A, Carson R, Bonne O, Lucnekbaugh D, et al. Reduced serotonin type 1_A receptor binding in panic disorder. Journal of Neuroscience. 2004;**24**:589-591. DOI: 10.1523/JNEUROSCI.4921-03.2004

[71] Isingrini E, Perret L, Rainer Q, Amilhon B, Guma E, Tanti A, et al. Resilience to chronic stress is mediated by noradrenergic regulation of dopamine neurons. Nature Neuroscience. 2016;**19**:560-563. DOI: 10.1038/nn.4245

[72] Kaye W, Jimerson D, Lake C, Ebert M. Altered norepinephrine metabolism following long-term weight recovery in patients with anorexia nervosa. Psychiatry Research. 1985;**14**:333-342. DOI: 10.1016/0165-1781(85)90101-5

[73] Kaye WH, Ebert MH, Raleigh M, Lake CR. Abnormalities in CNS monoamine metabolism in anorexia nervosa. Archives of General Psychiatry. 1984;**41**:350-355. DOI: 10.1001/archpsyc.1984.01790150040007

[74] Urwin RE, Bennetts B, Wilcken B, Lampropoulos B, Beumont P, Clarke S, et al. Anorexia nervosa (restrictive subtype) is associated with a polymorphism in the novel norepinephrine transporter gene promoter polymorphic region. Molecular Psychiatry. 2002;**7**:652-657. DOI: 10.1038/sj.mp.4001080

[75] Zucker NL, Herzog D, Moskovich A, Merwin R, Lin T. Incorporating dispositional traits into the treatment of anorexia nervosa. In: Adan RA, Kaye WH, editors. Behavioral Neurobiology of Eating Disorders. New York, NY: Springer; 2011. pp. 289-314

[76] Bernardoni F, King JA, Geisler D, Stein E, Jaite C, Nätsch D, et al. Weight restoration therapy rapidly reverses cortical thinning in anorexia nervosa: A longitudinal study. NeuroImage. 2016;**130**:214-222. DOI: 10.1016/j.neuroimage.2016.02.003

[77] Boghi A, Sterpone S, Sales S, D'Agata F, Bradac GB, Zullo G, et al. In vivo evidence of global and focal brain alterations in anorexia nervosa. Psychiatry Research: Neuroimaging. 2011;**192**:154-159. DOI: 10.1016/j.pscychresns.2010.12.008

[78] Kerem NC, Katzman DK. Brain structure and function in adolescents with anorexia nervosa. Adolescent Medicine Clinics. 2003;**14**:109-118

[79] Castro-Fornieles J, Bargalló N, Lazaro L, Andres S, Falcon C, Plana MT, et al. A cross-sectional and follow-up voxel-based morphometric MRI study in adolescent anorexia nervosa. Journal of Psychiatric Research. 2009;**43**:331-340. DOI: 10.1016/j.jpsychires.2008.03.013

[80] Joos A, Klöppel S, Hartmann A, Glauche V, Tüscher O, Perlov E, et al. Voxel-based morphometry in eating disorders: Correlation of psychopathology with grey matter volume. Psychiatry Research: Neuroimaging. 2010;**182**:146-151. DOI: 10.1016/j.pscychresns.2010.02.004

[81] Friederich HC, Walther S, Bendszus M, Biller A, Thomann P, Zeigermann S, et al. Grey matter abnormalities within cortico-limbic-striatal circuits in acute and weight-restored anorexia nervosa patients. NeuroImage. 2012;**59**:1106-1113. DOI: 10.1016/j.neuroimage.2011.09.042

[82] Gaudio S, Nocchi F, Franchin T, Genovese E, Cannatà V, Longo D, et al. Gray matter decrease distribution in the early stages of anorexia nervosa restrictive type in adolescents. Psychiatry Research: Neuroimaging. 2011;**191**:24-30. DOI: 10.1016/j.pscychresns.2010.06.007

[83] Seitz J, Buhren K, von Polier GG, Heussen N, Herpertz-Dahlmann B,

Konrad K. Morphological changes in the brain of acutely ill and weight-recovered patients with anorexia nervosa. A meta-analysis and qualitative review. Zeitschrift für Kinder- und Jugendpsychiatrie und Psychotherapie. 2014;**42**:7-17. DOI: 10.1024/1422-4917/a000265

[84] Mainz V, Schulte-Rüther M, Fink GR, Herpertz-Dahlmann B, Konrad K. Structural brain abnormalities in adolescent anorexia nervosa before and after weight recovery and associated hormonal changes. Psychosomatic Medicine. 2012;**74**:574-582. DOI: 10.1097/PSY.0b013e31824ef10e

[85] Roberto CA, Mayer LE, Brickman AM, Barnes A, Muraskin J, Yeung LK, et al. Brain tissue volume changes following weight gain in adults with anorexia nervosa. International Journal of Eating Disorders. 2011;**44**:406-411. DOI: 10.1002/eat.20840

[86] Rastam M, Bjure J, Vestergren E, Uvebrant P, Gillberg IC, Wentz E, et al. Regional cerebral blood flow in weight-restored anorexia nervosa: A preliminary study. Developmental Medicine & Child Neurology. 2001;**43**:239-242. DOI: 10.1111/j.1469-8749.2001.tb00196.x

[87] Cowdrey FA, Park RJ, Harmer CJ, McCabe C. Increased neural processing of rewarding and aversive food stimuli in recovered anorexia nervosa. Biological Psychiatry. 2011;**70**:736-743. DOI: 10.1016/j.biopsych.2011.05.028

[88] Santel S, Baving L, Krauel K, Munte T, Rotte M. Hunger and satiety in anorexia nervosa: fMRI during cognitive processing of food pictures. Brain Research. 2006;**1114**:138-148. DOI: 10.1016/j.brainres.2006.07.045

[89] Hinton E, Parkinson JA, Holland A, Arana F, Roberts A, Owen A. Neural contributions to the motivational control of appetite in humans. European Journal of Neuroscience. 2004;**20**:1411-1418. DOI: 10.1111/j.1460-9568.2004.03589.x

[90] Schoenfeld M, Neuer G, Tempelmann C, Schussler K, Noesselt T, Hopf J, et al. Functional magnetic resonance tomography correlates of taste perception in the human primary taste cortex. Neuroscience. 2004;**127**:347-353. DOI: 10.1016/j.neuroscience.2004.05.024

[91] Rolls ET. Taste, olfactory, and food texture processing in the brain, and the control of food intake. Physiology & Behavior. 2005;**85**:45-56. DOI: 10.1016/j.physbeh.2005.04.012

[92] Small D. Toward an understanding of the brain substrates of reward in humans. Neuron. 2002;**22**:668-671. DOI: 10.1016/S0896-6273(02)00620-7

[93] Kazama A, Bachevalier J. Selection aspiration of neurotoxic lesions of the orbitofrontal areas 11 and 13 spared monkey's performance on the object reversal discrimination task. Journal of Neuroscience. 2006;**29**:2794-2804. DOI: 10.1523/JNEUROSCI.4655-08.2009

[94] Clarke H, Walker SD, Robbins T, Roberts A. Cognitive inflexibility after prefrontal serotonin depletion is behaviorally and neurochemically specific. Cerebral Cortex. 2007;**17**:18-27. DOI: 10.1093/cercor/bhj120

[95] Fassino S, Pierò A, Gramaglia C, Abbate-Daga G. Clinical, psychopathological and personality correlates of interoceptive awareness in anorexia nervosa, bulimia nervosa and obesity. Psychopathology. 2004;**37**: 168-174. DOI: 10.1159/000079420

[96] Lilenfeld LR, Wonderlich S, Riso LP, Crosby R, Mitchell J. Eating disorders and personality: A methodological and empirical review. Clinical Psychology Review. 2006;**26**:299-320. DOI: 10.1016/j.cpr.2005.10.003

[97] Kaye WH, Wierenga CE, Bailer UF, Simmons AN, Bischoff-Grethe A. Nothing tastes as good as skinny feels: The neurobiology of anorexia nervosa. Trends in Neuroscience. 2013;**36**:110-120. DOI: 10.1016/j.tins.2013.01.003

[98] Nunn K, Frampton I, Gordon I, Lask B. The fault is not in her parents but in her insula—A neurobiological hypothesis of anorexia nervosa. European Eating Disorders Review. 2008;**16**:355-360. DOI: 10.1002/erv.890

[99] Bulik CM, Thornton LM, Root TL, Pisetsky EM, Lichtenstein P, Pedersen NL. Understanding the relation between anorexia nervosa and bulimia nervosa in a Swedish national twin sample. Biological Psychiatry. 2010;**67**:71-77. DOI: 10.1016/j.biopsych.2009.08.010

[100] Thornton LM, Mazzeo SE, Bulik CM. The heritability of eating disorders: Methods and current findings. In: Adan RA, Kaye WH, editors. Behavioral Neurobiology of Eating Disorders. New York, NY: Springer; 2011. pp. 141-156

[101] Uher R. The role of genetic variation in the causation of mental illness: An evolution-informed framework. Molecular Psychiatry. 2009;**14**:1072-1082. DOI: 10.1038/mp.2009.85

[102] Schaumberg K, Jangmo A, Thornton LM, Birgegård A, Almqvist C, Norring C, et al. Patterns of diagnostic transition in eating disorders: A longitudinal population study in Sweden. Psychological Medicine. 2018:1-9. DOI: 10.1017/S0033291718001472

[103] Bühren K, Schwarte R, Fluck F, Timmesfeld N, Krei M, Egberts K, et al. Comorbid psychiatric disorders in female adolescents with first-onset anorexia nervosa. European Eating Disorders Review. 2014;**22**:39-44. DOI: 10.1002/erv.2254

[104] Helder SG, Collier DA. The genetics of eating disorders. In: Adan RA, Kaye WH, editors. Behavioral Neurobiology of Eating Disorders. New York, NY: Springer; 2011. pp. 157-175

[105] Devlin B, Bacanu SA, Klump KL, Bulik CM, Fichter MM, Halmi KA, et al. Linkage analysis of anorexia nervosa incorporating behavioral covariates. Human Molecular Genetics. 2002;**11**:689-696. DOI: 10.1093/hmg/11.6.689

[106] Frieling H, Römer KD, Scholz S, Mittelbach F, Wilhelm J, De Zwaan M, et al. Epigenetic dysregulation of dopaminergic genes in eating disorders. International Journal of Eating Disorders. 2010;**43**:577-583. DOI: 10.1002/eat.20745

[107] Baker JH, Maes HH, Lissner L, Aggen SH, Lichtenstein P, Kendler KS. Genetic risk factors for disordered eating in adolescent males and females. Journal of Abnormal Psychology. 2009;**118**:576-586. DOI: 10.1037/a0016314

[108] Sloft-Op 't Landt MCT, Bartels M, Van Furth EF, Van Beijsterveldt CEM, Meulenbelt I, Slagboom PE, et al. Genetic influences on disordered eating behaviour are largely independent of body mass index. Acta Psychiatrica Scandinavica. 2008;**117**:348-356. DOI: 10.1111/j.1600-0447.2007.01132.x

[109] Klump KL, Burt SA, McGue M, Iacono WG. Changes in genetic and environmental influences on disordered eating across adolescence: A longitudinal twin study. Archives of General Psychiatry. 2007;**64**:1409-1415. DOI: 10.1001/archpsyc.64.12.1409

[110] Klump KL, Perkins PS, Burt SA, McGue MATT, Iacono WG. Puberty moderates genetic influences on disordered eating. Psychological Medicine. 2007;**37**:627-634. DOI: 10.1017/S0033291707000189

[111] Klump KL, Keel PK, Sisk C, Burt SA. Preliminary evidence that estradiol moderates genetic influences on disordered eating attitudes and behaviors during puberty. Psychological Medicine. 2010;**40**:1745-1753. DOI: 10.1017/S0033291709992236

[112] Bramen JE, Hranilovich JA, Dahl RE, Forbes EE, Chen J, Toga AW, et al. Puberty influences medial temporal lobe and cortical gray matter maturation differently in boys than girls matched for sexual maturity. Cerebral Cortex. 2011;**21**:636-646. DOI: 10.1093/cercor/bhq137

[113] Peper JS, Hulshoff Pol HE, Crone EA, van Honk J. Sex steroids and brain structure in pubertal boys and girls: A mini-review of neuroimaging studies. Neuroscience. 2011;**191**:28-37. DOI: 10.1016/j.neuroscience.2011.02.014

[114] Golden N, Carlson J. The pathophysiology of amenorrhea in the adolescent. Annals of the New York Academy of Sciences. 2008;1135: 163-178. DOI: 10.1196/annals.1429.014

[115] Chui HT, Christensen BK, Zipursky RB, Richards BA, Hanratty MK, Kabani NJ, et al. Cognitive function and brain structure in females with a history of adolescent-onset anorexia nervosa. Pediatrics. 2008;**122**:426-437. DOI: 10.1542/peds.2008-0170

Chapter 5

Possible Dysregulation of Orexin and Dopamine Systems in Anorexia Nervosa

Marcela Morales-Mulia and Sandra Morales-Mulia

Abstract

Anorexia nervosa (AN) is a psychiatric illness characterized by a lack of motivation and a taste for rewarding food consumption. Mood disorders such as depression and stress are frequently associated with this condition. Abnormalities in several neural systems have been identified in patients with AN, including serotonin, dopamine (DA), appetite-related neuropeptides, and other neurochemical systems. Moreover, the changes that occur between the mesolimbic dopaminergic pathway and the orexin neurons in the lateral hypothalamus (LH) in response to the reduction in food consumption are key in the development of AN. Several studies suggest a functional relationship between orexin and dopaminergic circuits. LH orexin neurons project dense fibers on dopaminergic neurons, potently activating these neurons. DA and orexin neurons regulate negative and positive motivational states, such as drug and food seeking behavior. For this reason, it is important to extend the study of the functional and emotional interactions that exist between both neuronal systems to design new drugs that act at a behavioral and molecular level to treat AN. This chapter provides an overview of the evidence from literature implicating dopamine-orexin systems in AN and discusses recent advances that have contributed to our current understanding of the mechanisms underlying the molecular bases of AN.

Keywords: mesocorticolimbic system, dopamine receptors, reward, mental illness, orexin neurons, motivation, anxiety disorders

1. Introduction

Anorexia nervosa (AN) has been classified as a chronic psychiatric disease since this condition has a strong emotional component. AN belongs to a group of eating disorders and is characterized by extreme body weight loss. AN patients show combination of physical, psychological, and behavioral disturbances that usually have their onset during adolescence. AN is associated with high levels of psychiatric comorbidity including psychosis, hyperactivity, depression, and anxiety. In consequence, this illness has become a major focus of attention in terms of both the research community and the general public. The prevalence of AN is approximately 1% in women and less than 0.5% in men [1]. Patients with AN show a high degree of anhedonia (the reduced capacity to experience reward or pleasure) and have a disturbed body image and an intense fear of weight gain. Standardized mortality ratios show that the rate of death in AN is at least five times greater than that in the general population [2].

Little is known about the etiology and the intrinsic biological alterations of anorexia, but it appears to be the result of different factors, for example, low self-esteem, certain personality traits such as perfectionism, mental illnesses such as depression, anxiety, self-harm, difficulty to manage stress and cope with life. Feelings of obsession and compulsion are also related with AN. Society and communication media play a key role in this pathology, since through them we are constantly told that the image of the body is very important because it reflects our value, as people. While culture, society, and the media exert pressure on women to remain thin, now it is widely accepted that there is a biological basis for this psychiatric disorder. Henceforth, the complexity of AN has limited the development of neuroscience-based treatments, and no medication or other biological treatment has been approved for the disorder. Then, to understand the biology of pathological eating behavior is an important step in the development of appropriate pharmacotherapies that can be used to treat AN patients.

To date abnormalities in several neural systems have been identified in patients with AN, including serotonin and DA, appetite-related neuropeptides, and other neurochemical systems. This chapter will focus especially on the dopaminergic neurons of the ventral tegmental area (VTA) that project the nucleus accumbens (NAc) to form the mesocorticolimbic circuit; and in the orexin neurons localized exclusively in two subregions of the hypothalamus; the perifornical area (PFA) and the LH, where orexin peptide is expressing [3].

Previously, it was thought that the serotonin system was the only or most important neurotransmitter involved in AN, and all research was carried out around its neurotransmission. Subsequently, preclinic and clinic evidence propose that the dopaminergic system could be a key factor in the pathophysiology of eating disorders. The AN is characterized by a reduction in food intake (diet restriction) and hyperactivity. In this sense, decrease in DA content has been observed in hypothalamus, hippocampus, and the dorsal striatum after a restricted diet. Moreover, the motor activity is modulated mainly by dopaminergic circuits. These first data point out for the first time the possible contribution of dopaminergic transmission in anorexia.

The signals to eat or to stop eating are very complex and extend beyond the control of the homeostatic system that responds to metabolic and satiety signals from the gut. Recently, it has been proposed that mesocorticolimbic dopaminergic system also responds to features of food such as the sight, smell, and taste in addition to cues that predict food intake and override the ingestive behavior [4]. The motivation to eat is key in eating behavior and is regulated by several intrinsic and extrinsic factors. Neuronal and circulating peptides are released in response of internal states, such as hunger or satiety, to stimulate or repress food intake, respectively. Accumulating evidence has pointing out the orexin-containing neurons as central regulators of feeding behavior, energy balance modulation, and metabolic homeostasis.

2. Dopamine neurons

DA is a catecholamine and is a key neuromodulator involved in motivated behaviors. DA-containing neurons are characterized by the presence of tyrosine hydroxylase (TH), the rate-limiting enzyme in the synthesis of catecholamines, and are found throughout the mammalian central nervous system (CNS), including the ventral midbrain (VM) [5]. Midbrain DA-containing neurons are arranged principally in two nucleus: the substantia nigra pars compacta (SNc, also known as the A9 group) and the VTA, or A10 group [5, 6]. Different populations of DA-containing neurons project to distinct areas and control or modulate specific functions, according to their targets. We will emphasize in the VTA nucleus, which project to ventromedial striatum (NAc) and PFC, forming the mesocorticolimbic system. These DA-containing neurons regulate emotional behavior, natural motivation, reward and cognitive function, and are largely implicated in a range of psychiatric disorders [7–9].

DA acts primly through of two G protein-coupled DA D1 (D1R) and D2 (D2R) receptors [10]. D1R is a postsynaptic receptor that mediates more directly behavior, and the D2R is a presynaptic autoreceptor that regulates DA release in a negative feedback fashion; D1R increases, whereas D2R decreases adenylyl-cyclase activity, and both receptor types are distributed throughout the CNS [11]. A variety of studies indicate that an altered DA function in AN could be implicated. Patients with AN have shown low levels of homovanillic acid in their cerebrospinal fluid (CSF), the major DA metabolite [12]; in addition, a positron emission tomography (PET) study revealed an increase in D2R binding in the anteroventral striatum (NAc in rodents), in a mixed group of women recovered from both restricted-type anorexia nervosa and binge-eating/purging-type [13]. These data suggest that neuronal or synaptic DA may be reduced, but that DA receptors could be increased in number or sensitivity in a compensatory or negative feedback fashion [14]. Thus, a down-regulation of receptor sensitivity might be an important therapeutic goal in AN, to compensate the low levels of DA.

Several hypotheses have been raised about the contribution of DA in AN. On one side, Bergh and Södersten [15] suggest that normal DA responses to hunger and exercise facilitate a progression into AN; in addition, O'Hara et al. [16] proposed that an anomaly in the reward system mediated by the DA leads to the development, maintenance, and resistance to the treatment of the AN.

2.1 Mesocorticolimbic dopamine neurons may facilitate the development of anorexia nervosa

According to Bergh and Södersten [15], dieting, along with high levels of exercise, leads to a stress response that increases cortisol and corticotrophin-releasing factor (CRF) [17–22], which in turn promotes an increase in DA levels in the NAc [23, 24]. In such a way, DA facilitates rewarding behaviors such as diet and exercise to become habits similar to those associated with drug dependency or self-starvation by conditioning this type of reward to initially neutral stimuli [15, 25–28]. In addition, the high CRF levels induced by diet restriction and exercise also facilitate to seek for food, while simultaneously suppressing food intake [29]. However, until now there is no clinical study that compares the DA levels in anorexic subjects before and after developing anorexia that shows chronically high levels of DA before the disease was declared.

2.2 Aberrant concept of starvation in anorexia nervosa

The mentalistic concept of AN assumes that it results from a mental illness. This concept describes this illness as a set of chronic and serious mental disorders with debilitating physical, cognitive, and socioemotional impairments such as anxiety, depression, obsessional traits, and pathological cognitions. Therefore, when the initial care of a patient with anorexia is focused only on cognitive therapies to treat psychological disorders do not usually give good long-time results. Moreover, symptoms such as anxiety and depression also emerge in healthy people during a starvation period [30]. There are many arguments against the hypothesis that an underlying mental disorder causes AN [31]. Recently, it was discovered that AN and anxiety have different genetic risk factors. Also, almost all mental disorder symptoms observed in anorexics disappear after normalization of eating behavior [31, 32].

O'Hara et al. [16] do not agree with the mentalist concept because this does not assume the normal functions of the neuroendocrine system, which is responsible for regulating the release of peptides that regulate food consumption. The mentalist concept does not take into account the physiological aspects in eating disorders, and this may be the reason why this approach to treating anorexia as a consequence of a mental illness has not led to an effective treatment. O'Hara et al. [16] proposed that an abnormality in the reward system mediated by DA leads to the development, maintenance, and resistance to treatment in the AN.

They suggest that the decrease in dopaminergic activity and the rejection of food intake are key in the development of anorexia. Therefore, they propose increasing DA levels to normalize the consumption of food to reduce the stress generated by starvation, which in turn reduces the release of CRF to gradually increase the consumption of food. However, recent studies suggest that changes in DA found in anorexic patients are due more to a normal characteristic of starvation than to a disease marker.

3. Hypothalamic orexin neurons modulate dopaminergic neurons

Orexin-A and orexin-B neuropeptides were initially identified as endogenous ligands for two orphan G protein-coupled receptors; the OX_1R is coupled entirely to Gq, whereas OX_2R is coupled to both Gi/o and Gq [33]. Both orexins are derived from proteolytic cleavage, of a precursor peptide (pre-pro-orexin), and are produced by a group of neurons in the LH and PFA, a region known as the feeding center (**Figure 1**). OX-A has the same affinity with both receptors, while OX-B has a greater affinity for OX_2R than OX_1R [33, 34]. These receptors are highly expressed throughout the brain including the "dopaminergic reward pathways" (**Figure 1**) [35–39]. Moreover, these

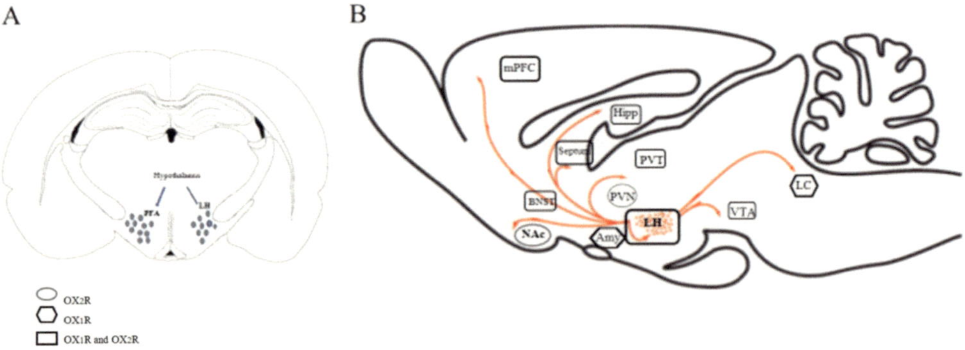

Figure 1.
Schematic representation of the brain areas related to motivated and emotional behaviors. (A) Coronal section of the rat brain showing the lateral (LH) and perifornical area (PEA) of hypothalamus. (B) Representation of the main orexin projections and the expression of orexin receptors 1 and 2 (OX_1R and OX_2R) in these brain regions. The fear circuit comprising the hippocampus (Hypp), medial prefrontal cortex (mPFC), and amygdala (AMY). Areas implicated in anxiety: bed of the stria terminals (BNST), paraventricular thalamus (PVT), and septum. The paraventricular nucleus of the hypothalamus (PVN) regulates stress responses and the hypothalamic-pituitary-adrenal axis hormone cascade. The mesocorticolimbic system modulates the rewarding properties of food and drugs of abuse and comprising the ventral tegmental area (VTA) and nucleus accumbens (NAc). The locus coeruleus (LC) also has dense orexin innervations in concordance with its involvement in arousal and emotional memory. Abbreviation: LH, lateral hypothalamus.

peptides are also regarded as an important factor that regulates feeding behavior, owing to their localization within the lateral hypothalamic area, the classic "feeding center."

Orexins were recognized as positive regulators of energy expenditure, thanks to the development of the orexin neuron-deficient mice. Studies conducted in these animals led to propose that orexins promote acute food consumption on one hand and on the other hand prevent the progress of obesity [40]. Since then, numerous pharmacological and genetic studies have supported that these peptides together with their receptors are key regulators of energy expenditure, thus influencing the energy balance.

The activation of the orexin system by means of the microinjection of orexin-A in the hypothalamus has shown that these peptides act as protectors in the development of obesity, by increasing energy expenditure. Also, orexin neurons increase energy expenditure by increasing thermogenesis in brown adipose tissue [40]. On the other hand, it has been observed that overexoression of pre-pro-orexin gene in an animal model promotes resistance to obesity induced by consumption of a high-fat diet [41]

The available anatomical, genetic, and pharmacological evidence supports that the behavioral consequences of the activity of the orexin system are due to parallel signaling to multiple brain regions and neurotransmitter systems such as DA. For example, the NAc is involved in hedonic and motivational aspects of feeding [42] and is an important brain region because endogenous orexin peptides act to modulate DA release [43], which act over hedonic processes associated with food evaluation and consumption. In addition, NAc is involved in the reward of natural behaviors, such as exercise, sex, and, of course food intake.

Orexins in the VTA, the major dopaminergic nucleus, have been implicated in drug and alcohol seeking and reinstatement. as well as food seeking, in highly salient circumstances, food seeking in highly salient circumstances, for example, during hunger, presentation of palatable foods or with exposure to food-related cues, but not in the consumption of regular food [44, 45]. An alternative mechanism by which orexins can stimulate the consumption of highly palatable food is via the paraventricular thalamic nucleus (PVT) because orexin neurons in the hypothalamus also send dense projections to the PVT [37], which in turn regulates DA efflux to the NAc via its glutamatergic projections [46, 47]. It has been reported that orexin actions in PVT promote DA efflux in the NAc, while the inhibition of its receptor OX_1R in this region decreases hedonic intake of palatable foods [48]. Therefore, orexins not only can act directly in the VTA to increase DA [45, 49] but they also increase DA via action in the PVT to promote hedonic food intake [48]. In summary, the control that orexins exert over VTA-NAc circuit is key to modulate motivational behaviors and reward processes related to drug, alcohol, and food seeking.

Functional studies show the relationship between LH orexins and VTA-NAc circuit where orexins exert their actions on the dopaminergic neurons by increasing the firing frequency in VTA neurons in vitro and in vivo [50, 51]. These peptides induce an increase in DA release and its metabolites in both NAc and PFC [4, 49, 52, 53]. Electrical stimulation of the LH nucleus can increase both food intake and accumbal DA turnover [54–56]. In contrast, the inhibition of OX1R reduces DA cells firing [57], as well as significantly decrease in amphetamine, and cocaine-induced DA release in the NAc [57, 58]. On the other hand, the intracerebroventricular administration of OX-A leads to stress-related behavior like grooming, stereotypy, and hyperlocomotion [59], actions that were inhibited by DA D1 receptor (D1R) or DA D2 receptor (D2R) antagonists in rodents [59]. These data provide strong evidence that the orexin system contributes to DAergic neurons regulation in the mesocorticolimbic pathway and that the action of orexins in these neurons could involve a variety of behaviors that are known to be regulated by DA.

This framework suggests that understanding the function of the orexin requires studying them in a brain region-specific basis, as well as understanding the interactions between different brain regions that receive orexinergic input [40]

4. Anorexia nervosa and anxiety disorders: role of orexin and dopamine

4.1 Anorexia nervosa and anxiety disorders

AN is a very complex disease, characterized by a profound dysregulation in neurocircuits related to control eating behavior, anxiety, fear, and reward positive/negative reinforcers. AN is a serious motivated behavioral condition with high morbidity and mortality. Anorexic patients usually have a high comorbidity with severe anxiety disorders, such as obsessive-compulsive disorder (OCD) and social anxiety disorder (SAD) [60]. One characteristic that anorexics share with people suffering from SAD is their fear and concern about how other people perceive them. Elevated neuroticism and perfectionism as well as decreased novelty seeking are anxious personality traits observed in these disorders [60]. Therefore, anxiety disorders and AN are strongly correlated; in both disorders, the fear is organized around an irrational belief associated with heightened vigilance and pronounced anxiety. Another characteristic shared between AN and OCD is compulsivity: to engage in repetitive and stereotyped acts that have unwanted outcomes [61] and arises from a reduced ability to control inflexible yet maladaptive behavior as the starvation, which persists in the face of negative consequences, for example, interfering with academic/occupational/social interests in longer term and the behaviors promoting further, and potentially dangerous, weight loss.

Recently, Lloyd et al. [62] have proposed a central role for anxiety in the development of compulsive starvation; they suggest a dual mechanism by which anxiety could be motivating the initiation of AN and propose that the reinforcement effects of starvation cause excessive repetition of behaviors leading to the buildout of psychological symptoms of AN. They also suggest that starvation becomes compulsive until it has adverse implications for anxiety, which generates the symptoms of AN and which encourages the formation of a vicious circle that guarantees the persistence of an extreme dietary restriction. Stress and distress tolerance have been suggested as important factors in determining the onset and course of AN [61]. Stressful and traumatic events often precede eating diseases. Notably, high levels of anxiety tend to also precede the onset of addiction and OCD.

Dietary restriction has an anxiolytic effect, because women recovered from AN show elevated levels of serotonin (5-HT) metabolites [63], and gene variants linked to more active 5-HT and noradrenaline (NA) systems are implicated in AN [64, 65], supporting the involvement of these neurotransmitter systems in the heightened anxiety that precedes AN. Thus, dietary restriction relieves the anxiety (or negative reinforcement) provided by the dietary restriction that increases with anxiety.

Starvation is a compulsive behavior that over time becomes a habit with a dominant influence in individuals with AN. Surprisingly, in anorexics, there is an imperative need to keep starving [62]. However, this behavior puts your life at risk.

Subjects with AN show an extreme aversive state characterized by high levels of anxiety when eating, that is, when they do not carry out their compulsive behavior of starvation [61, 66]. This is also observed in addiction and OCD, where the execution of compulsions serves to temporarily relieve the negative effects [61, 67–69].

Several studies indicate that the levels of anxiety in anorexics are even higher than before the restriction of food and that this anxious behavior is partially mediated by an increased sensitivity of the 5-HT and NA systems, which results from the reduced consumption of tryptophan and tyrosine, respectively [70, 71].

When starvation becomes necessary to avoid an extremely anxious state, the desire to starve is enhanced given the poor emotion regulation abilities of individuals with AN, which limits the use of alternative strategies to overcome dysphoria [72–74].

Anxiety precedes and coincides with restrictive eating in AN [75–78], which is not the case for individuals without the disorder [77]. Repeatedly engaging in dietary restriction in an anxious state facilitates anxiety to evoke restrictive eating habits, due to a pairing of emotion and behavior.

Thus, several mechanisms likely explain how anxiety promotes engagement in maladaptive dietary restriction habits that have developed during a compulsive illness.

4.2 Dopamine and orexins systems: evidence for an interconnection in anorexia nervosa

Stress and distress tolerance have been suggested as important factors in determining the onset and course of AN. Stressful and traumatic events often precede eating diseases. AN comprises a hyperactivation of the HPA axis [79]. Patients with AN present significantly elevated concentration of plasma cortisol, increased central CRF, and significantly less cortisol suppression after dexamethasone administration than controls [80, 81]. Moreover, hormonal changes also do not seem to be specific for AN and are found in other diseases or in healthy subjects as a consequence of malnutrition and starvation [82]. In general, these data show the need to study other molecules as possible indicators of HPA-axis hyperactivity on the one hand and that regulate emotional states on the other hand. DA and orexins share diverse characteristics at the physiological, psychological, and psychiatric levels, such as the ability to modulate the HPA axis activity, induce drug and food seeking behavior, increase the motivation to obtain food, and regulate emotional states, such as depression and anxiety.

At first it was thought that orexins participated in the consumption of food because orexin central administration produces food seeking, and food deprivation increases orexin mRNA [83, 84]. In addition, orexin neurons are excited by peripheral signals of nutrient needs (e.g., ghrelin), inhibited by satiety signals (e.g., glucose) and interact with feeding peptides to promote food consumption and seeking [85–89]. Notably, orexin neurons are active during hunger and help to translate peripheral hunger signals into increased appetitive responding for food and cues associated to consumption of food. Thus, orexins facilitate food seeking especially in motivationally charged circumstances.

Orexins orchestrate various aspects of stress responses. For example, acute (but not chronic and predictable) stress is associated with orexin neuron activation [90]. The orexins help to organize the response to stress, but only when it assumes a motivated and adaptable behavior to cope with stress, that is, when you can escape the stressor. In contrast, when a stressor is chronic, predictable, and impossible to escape, the activity of orexin system decreases, and this hypoactivity can produce motivational symptoms similar to depression.

In the case of DA, it is involved in motivational but not consummatory aspects of feeding. The blocking of mesocorticolimbic dopaminergic system decreases the response for motivational tasks associated with obtaining food [91]. DA depletion or administration of DA receptor antagonists in NAc reduces the motivation to consumption high palatable food [92–95]. The motivation to eat is a key factor to maintain a normal feeding behavior.

Dysfunction of the OXs and DA systems may contribute to the pathology of anxiety and addiction to food and drugs of abuse, which is commonly associated with anxiety and/or defective fear processing, depression, and cognitive impairment as well as other comorbid conditions. Increase in orexin mRNA levels has been observed in animals exposed to different stressors such as immobilization [96], cold stress [96], or hypoglycemia [84], while that both acute and chronic stress promote major changes in DA signaling in the mesocorticolimbic pathway such as increases in DA release in the striatum, NAc, and PFC [97–99]. D2R receptor knockout mice display anxiety and depression-like behaviors upon chronic stress [100]. Repeated restrain stress produces increases and decreases in DA receptor densities within the mesoaccumbens and nigrostriatal systems in two different strains of mice [101]. So, these results suggested that stressful conditions could be augmented the vulnerability to develop psychiatric illnesses as AN. So, any decline in the transmission of DA and orexins can generate a lack of motivation to consume food. However, there are few studies about the participation of DA receptors in the PFA/HL areas on the control of food drinking. Studies suggest that ethanol intake and excessive food consumption could be similarly affected by DA in the PFA/HL areas, with increases in both ethanol and food intake after D1 receptor activation and decrease in both consumptions after the activation of D2 [100].

Considering that the anxiety induces specific reduction of the D2R in the NAc and that DA attenuates several addictive behaviors in animals [100], it is difficult not to think that DA may act as an anxiolytic agent through the D2R activation. On the other hand, the decreased release of orexins could promote low food consumption, that is, the dysfunction of the orexin system could be accentuating the lack of motivation for the search and consumption of food in anorexics. In this way, the stimulation of orexin receptors together with DA could reduce the stress generated by starvation and, at the same time, increase the motivation for food consumption.

5. Conclusion

Considering on the one hand that AN is a compulsive disorder, and on the other hand that starvation is the result of a negative reinforcement, it is suggested that the dysfunction of DA and orexins in the mesocorticolimbic system is key to the successful treatment of AN. The model can justify the use of existing and planned prevention and treatment programs but may also guide the development of novel interventions to favorably affect the incidence and recovery rates of a life-threatening condition.

Acknowledgements

To the Consejo Nacional de Ciencia y Tecnología (CONACyT 241216) and Instituto Nacional de Psiquiatría Ramón de la Fuente Muñiz (IC16033.0).

Conflict of interest

The authors declare that they have no conflict of interest.

Nomenclature

AN	anorexia nervosa
HPA axis	hypothalamic-pituitary-adrenal axis
CNS	central nervous system
CRF	corticotrophin-releasing factor
DA	dopamine
D1R	dopamine D1 receptor
D2R	dopamine D2 receptor
LH	lateral hypothalamus
mRNA	messenger ribonucleic acid
NA	noradrenaline
NAc	nucleus accumbens
OCD	obsessive-compulsive disorder
OX_1R	orexin 1 receptor
OX_2R	orexin 2 receptor
PVT	paraventricular thalamic nucleus
PFA	perifornical area
5-HT	serotonin
SAD	social anxiety disorder
SNc	substantia nigra pars compacta
TH	tyrosine hydroxylase
VM	ventral midbrain
VTA	ventral tegmental area

Author details

Marcela Morales-Mulia[1*] and Sandra Morales-Mulia[2]

1 National Institute of Psychiatry RFM, Mexico City, Mexico

2 Science Faculty, Autonomous University of Mexico, UNAM, Mexico City, Mexico

*Address all correspondence to: mmulia@imp.edu.mx

References

[1] Zipfel S, Giel KE, Bulik CM, Hay P, Schmidt U. Anorexia nervosa: Aetiology, assessment, and treatment. Lancet Psychiatry. Dec 2015;**2**(12):1099-1111. DOI: 10.1016/S2215-0366(15)00356-9

[2] Arcelus J, Mitchell AJ, Wales J, Nielsen S. Mortality rates in patients with anorexia nervosa and other eating disorders. A meta-analysis of 36 studies. Archives of General Psychiatry. Jul 2011;**68**(7):724-731. DOI: 10.1001/archgenpsychiatry.2011.74

[3] Yoshida K, McCormack S, España RA, Crocker A, Scammell TE. Afferents to the orexin neurons of the rat brain. Journal of Comparative Neurology. 2006;**494**:845-861. DOI: 10.1002/cne.20859

[4] Palmiter RD. Is dopamine a physiologically relevant mediator of feeding behavior? Trends in Neurosciences. 2007;**30**:375-381. DOI: 10.1016/j.tins.2007.06.004

[5] Björklund A, Hökfelt T. Handbook of Chemical Neuroanatomy. Elsevier: Amsterdam; New York; 1983

[6] Dahlström A, Fuxe K. Localization of monoamines in the lower brain stem. Experientia. 1964;**20**:398-399

[7] Carlsson ML. On the role of prefrontal cortex glutamate for the antithetical phenomenology of obsessive compulsive disorder and attention deficit hyperactivity disorder. Progress in Neuropsychopharmacology & Biological Psychiatry. 2001;**25**:5-26. DOI: 10.1016/S0278-5846(00)00146-9

[8] Chao J, Nestler EJ. Molecular neurobiology of drug addiction. Annual Review of Medicine. 2004;**55**:113-132. DOI: 10.1146/annurev.med.55.091902.103730

[9] Hornykiewicz O. Psychopharmacological implications of dopamine and dopamine antagonists: A critical evaluation of current evidence. Neuroscience. 1978;**3**:773-783. DOI: 10.1016/0306-4522(78)90030-1

[10] Asakawa A, Inui A, Momose K, Ueno N, Fujino MA, Kasuga M. Endomorphins have orexigenic and anxiolytic activities in mice. Neuroreport. 1998;**9**:2265-2267

[11] Cooper JR, Bloom FE, Roth RH. The Biochemical Basis of Neuropharmacology. 8th ed. Oxford: Oxford University Press; 2003. 518 p. DOI: 10.1093/ageing/afw180

[12] Kaye WH, Ebert MH, Raleigh M, Lake R. Abnormalities in CNS monoamine metabolism in anorexia nervosa. Archives of General Psychiatry. 1984;**41**:350-355. DOI: 10.1176/ajp.141.12.1598

[13] Frank GK, Bailer UF, Henry SE, Drevets W, Meltzer CC, Price JC, et al. Increased dopamine D2/D3 receptor binding after recovery from anorexia nervosa measured by positron emission tomographyand [11c]raclopride. Biological Psychiatry. 2005;**58**:908-912. DOI: 10.1016/j.biopsych.2005.05.003

[14] Karson CN. Spontaneous eye-blink rates and dopaminergic systems. Brain. 1983;**106**:643-653

[15] Bergh C, Södersten P. Anorexia nervosa, self-starvation and the reward of stress. Nature Medicine. 1996;**2**:21-22

[16] O'Hara CB, Campbell IC, Schmidt U. A reward-centred model of anorexia nervosa: A focussed narrative review of the neurological and psychophysiological literature. Neuroscience & Biobehavioral. Reviews.

2015;**52**:131-152. DOI: 10.1016/j.neubiorev.2015.02.012

[17] Hotta M, Shibasaki T, Masuda A, Imaki T, Demura H, Ling N, et al. The responses of plasma adrenocorticotropin and cortisol to corticotropin-releasing hormone (CRH) and cerebrospinal fluid immunoreactive CRH in anorexia nervosa patients. Journal of Clinical Endocrinology and Metabolism. 1986;**62**:319-324. DOI: 10.1210/jcem-62-2-319

[18] Rojo L, Conesa L, Bermudez O, Livianos L. Influence of stress in the onset of eating disorders: Data from a two-stage epidemiologic controlled study. Psychosomatic Medicine. 2006;**68**:628-635. DOI: 10.1097/01.psy.0000227749.58726.41

[19] Estour B, Germain N, Diconne E, Frere D, Cottet-Emard J-M, Carrot G, et al. Hormonal profile heterogeneity and short-term physical risk in restrictive anorexia nervosa. Journal of Clinical Endocrinology & Metabolism. 2010;**95**:2203-2210. DOI: 10.1210/jc.2009-2608

[20] Gwirtsman HE, Kaye WH, George DT, Jimerson DC, Ebert MH, Gold PW. Central and peripheral ACTH and cortisol levels in anorexia nervosa and bulimia. Archives of General Psychiatry. 1989;**46**:61-69. DOI: 10.1001/archpsyc.1989.01810010063009

[21] Schorr M, Lawson EA, Dichtel LE, Klibanski A, Miller KK. Cortisol measures across the weight spectrum. Journal of Clinical Endocrinology & Metabolism. 2015;**100**:3313-3321. DOI: 10.1210/JC.2015-2078

[22] Shibuya I, Nagamitsu S, Okamura H, Komatsu H, Ozono S, Yamashita Y, et al. Changes in salivary cortisol levels as a prognostic predictor in children with anorexia nervosa. International Journal of Psychophysiology. Nov 2011;**82**(2):196-201. DOI: 10.1016/j.ijpsycho.2011.08.008

[23] Holly EN, DeBold JF, Miczek KA. Increased mesocorticolimbic dopamine during acute and repeated social defeat stress: Modulation by corticotropin releasing factor receptors in the ventral tegmental area. Psychopharmacology. 2015;**232**:4469-4479. DOI: 10.1007/s00213-015-4082-z

[24] Wanat MJ, Hopf FW, Stuber GD, Phillips PE, Bonci A. Corticotropin-releasing factor increases mouse ventral tegmental area dopamine neuron firing through a protein kinase C-dependent enhancement of Ih. Journal of Physiology. 2008;**586**(8):2157-2170. DOI: 10.1113/jphysiol.2007

[25] Everitt BJ, Robbins TW. Neural systems of reinforcement for drug addiction: From actions to habits to compulsion. Nature Neuroscience. 2005;**8**:1481-1489. DOI: 10.1038/nn1579

[26] Jansen A. A learning model of binge eating: Cue reactivity and cue exposure. Behaviour Research and Therapy. 1998;**36**:257-272. DOI: 10.1016/S0005-7967(98)00055-2

[27] Méquinion M, Chauveau C, Viltart O. The use of animal models to decipher physiological and neurobiological alterations of anorexia nervosa patients. Frontiers in Endocrinology (Lausanne). 2015;**6**:68. DOI: 10.3389/fendo.2015.00068

[28] Södersten P, Nergårdh R, Bergh C, Zandian M, Scheurink A. Behavioral neuroendocrinology and treatment of anorexia nervosa. Frontiers in Neuroendocrinology. 2008;**29**:445-462. DOI: 10.1016/j.yfrne.2008.06.001

[29] Stengel A, Taché Y. CRF and urocortin peptides as modulators of energy balance and feeding behavior during stress. Frontiers in

Neuroscience. 2014;**8**:52. DOI: 10.3389/fnins.2014.00052

[30] Keys A, Brozek J, Henschel A, Mickelsen O, Taylor HL. The Biology of Human Starvation. Minneapolis, MN: University of Minnesota Press; 1950

[31] Bergh C, Callmar M, Danemar S, Hölcke M, Isberg S, Leon M, et al. Effective treatment of eating disorders: Results at multiple sites. Behavioral Neuroscience. 2013;**127**:878-889. DOI: 10.1037/a0034921

[32] Bergh C, Brodin U, Lindberg G, Södersten P. Randomized controlled trial of a treatment for anorexia and bulimia nervosa. Proceedings of the National Academy of Sciences of the United States of America. 2002;**99**:9486-9491. DOI: 10.1073/pnas.142284799

[33] Zhu Y, Miwa Y, Yamanaka A, Yada T, Shibahara M, Abe Y, et al. Orexin receptor type-1 couples exclusively to pertussis toxin-insensitive G-proteins, while orexin receptor type-2 couples to both pertussis toxin-sensitive and –insensitive G-proteins. Journal of Pharmaceutical Sciences. 2003;**92**:259-266. DOI: 10.1254/jphs.92.259

[34] Suzuki M, Beuckmann CT, Shikata K, Ogura H, Sawai T. Orexin-A (hipocretins-1) is possibly involved in generation of anxiety-like behavior. Brain Research. 2005;**1044**:116-121. DOI: 10.1016/j.brainres.2005.03.002

[35] Carelli RM. Nucleus accumbens cell firing during goal-directed behaviors for cocaine vs. 'natural' reinforcement. Physiology & Behavior. 2002;**76**:379-387. DOI: 10.1016/S0031-9384(02)00760-6

[36] Koob GF, Bloom FE. Cellular and molecular mechanisms of drug dependence. Science. 1988;**242**:715-723. DOI: 10.1126/science.2903550

[37] Peyron C, Tighe DK, van den Pol AN, de Lecea L, Heller HC, Sutcliffe JG, et al. Neurons containing hypocretin (orexin) project to multiple neuronal systems. Journal of Neuroscience. 1998;**18**:9996-10015. DOI: 10.1523/JNEUROSCI.18-23-09996

[38] Sutcliffe JG, de Lecea L. The hypocretins: Setting the arousal threshold. Nature Review Neuroscience. 2002;**3**:339-349. DOI: 10.1038/nrn808

[39] Wise RA, Rompre PP. Brain dopamine and reward. Annual Review of Psychology. 1989;**40**:191-225. DOI: 10.1146/annurev.ps.40.020189.001203

[40] Perez-Leighton1 CE, Butterick-Peterson TA, Billington CJ, Kotz CM. Role of orexin receptors in obesity: From cellular to behavioral evidence. International Journal of Obesity. 2013;**37**:167-174. DOI: 10.1038/ijo.2012.30

[41] Funato H, Tsai AL, Willie JT, Kisanuki Y, Williams SC, Sakurai T, et al. Enhanced orexin receptor-2 signaling prevents diet-induced obesity and improves leptin sensitivity. Cell Metabolism. 2009;**9**:64-76. DOI: 10.1016/j.cmet.2008.10.010

[42] Wise RA. Role of brain dopamine in food reward and reinforcement. Philosophical Transactions of the Royal Society London B: Biological Sciences. 2006;**361**:1149-1158. DOI: 10.1098/rstb.2006.1854

[43] Narita M, Nagumo Y, Miyatake M, Ikegami D, Kurahashi K, Suzuki T. Implication of protein kinase C in the orexin-induced elevation of extracellular dopamine levels and its rewarding effect. European Journal of Neuroscience. 2007;**25**:1537-1545. DOI: 10.1111/j.1460-9568.2007.05403.x

[44] Borgland SL, Chang S-J, Bowers MS, Thompson JL, Vittoz N, Floresco SB, et al. Orexin A/hypocretin-1 selectively

promotes motivation for positive reinforcers. Journal of Neuroscience. 2009;**29**:11215-11225. DOI: 10.1523/JNEUROSCI.6096-08.2009

[45] España RA, Oleson EB, Locke JL, Brookshire BR, Roberts DC, Jones SR. The hypocretin–orexin system regulates cocaine self-administration via actions on the mesolimbic dopamine system. European Journal of Neuroscience. 2010;**31**:336-348. DOI: 10.1111/j.1460-9568.2009.07065.x

[46] Jones MW, Kilpatrick IC, Phillipson OT. Regulation of dopamine function in the nucleus accumbens of the rat by the thalamic paraventricular nucleus and adjacent midline nuclei. Experimentral Brain Research. 1989;**76**:572-580

[47] Parsons MP, Li S, Kirouac GJ. Functional and anatomical connection between the paraventricular nucleus of the thalamus and dopamine fibers of the nucleus accumbens. Journal of Comparative Neurology. 2007;**500**:1050-1063. DOI: 10.1002/cne.21224

[48] Choi DL, Davis JF, Magrisso IJ, Fitzgerald ME, Lipton JW, Benoit SC. Orexin signaling in the paraventricular thalamic nucleus modulates mesolimbic dopamine and hedonic feeding in the rat. Neuroscience. 2012;**210**:243-248. DOI: 10.1016/j.neuroscience.2012.02.036

[49] Vittoz NM, Berridge CW. Hypocretin/orexin selectively increases dopamine efflux within the prefrontal cortex: Involvement of the ventral tegmental area. Neuropsychopharmacology. 2006;**31**:384-395. DOI: 10.1038/sj.npp.1300807

[50] Korotkova TM, Sergeeva OA, Eriksson KS, Haas HL, Brown RE. Excitation of ventral tegmental area dopaminergic and nondopaminergic neurons by orexins/hypocretins. Journal of Neuroscience. 2003;**23**:7-11. DOI: 10.1523/JNEUROSCI.23-01-00007.2003

[51] Muschamp JW, Dominguez JM, Sato SM, Shen RY, Hull EM. A role for hypocretin (orexin) in male sexual behavior. Journal of Neuroscience. 2007;**27**:2837-2845. DOI: 10.1523/JNEUROSCI.4121-06.2007

[52] España RA, Melchior JR, Roberts DC, Jones SR. Hypocretin 1/orexin A in the ventral tegmental area enhances dopamine responses to cocaine and promotes cocaine self-administration. Psychopharmacology. 2011;**214**:415-426. DOI: 10.1007/s00213-010-2048-8

[53] Vittoz NM, Schmeichel B, Berridge CW. Hypocretin/orexin preferentially actives caudomedial ventral tegmental areas dopamine neurons. European Journal of Neuroscience. 2008;**28**:1629-1640. DOI: 10.1111/j.1460-9568.2008.06453.x

[54] Hernandez L, Hoebel BG. Feeding and hypothalamic stimulation increase dopamine turnover in the accumbens. Physiology & Behavior. 1988;**44**:599-606. DOI: 10.1016/0031-9384(88)90324-1

[55] Hoebel BG, Hernandez L, Schwartz DH, Mark GP, Hunter GA. Microdialysis studies of brain norepinephrine, serotonin, and dopamine release during ingestive behavior. Theoretical and clinical implications. Annals of the New York Academy of Sciences. 1989;**575**:171-193. DOI: 10.1111/j.1749-6632.1989.tb53242.x

[56] Moorman DE, Aston-Jones G. Orexin/hypocretin modulates response of ventral tegmental dopamine neurons to prefrontal activation: Diurnal influences. Journal of Neuroscience. 2010;**30**:15585-15599. DOI: 10.1523/JNEUROSCI.2871-10.2010

[57] Prince CD, Rau AR, Yorgason JT, España RA. Hypocretin/orexin

regulation of dopamine signaling and cocaine self-administration is mediated predominantly by hypocretin receptor 1. ACS Chemical Neuroscience. 2015;**21**:138-146. DOI: 10.1021/cn500246j

[58] Quarta D, Valerio E, Hutchenson DM, Hedou G, Heidbreder C. The orexin-1 receptor antagonists SB-334867 reduce amphetamine-evoked dopamine outflow in the shell of the nucleus accumbens and decreases the expression of amphetamine sensitization. Neurochemistry International. 2010;**56**:11-15. DOI: 10.1016/j.neuint.2009.08.012

[59] Nakamura T, Uramura K, Nambu T, Yada T, Goto K, Yanagisawa M, et al. Orexin-induced hyperlocomotion and stereotypy are mediated by the dopaminergic system. Brain Research. 2000;**873**:181-187. DOI: 10.1016/S0006-8993(00)02555-5

[60] Guarda AS, Schreyer CC, Boersma GJ, Tamashiro KL, Moran TH. Anorexia nervosa as a motivated behavior: Relevance of anxiety, stress, fear and learning. Physiology & Behavior. 2015;**152**:466-472. DOI: 10.1016/j.physbeh.2015.04.007

[61] Fineberg NA, Menchon JM, Zohar J, Veltman DJ. Compulsivity—A new trans-diagnostic research domain for the roadmap for mental Health Research in Europe (ROAMER) and research domain criteria (RDoC) initiatives. European Neuropsychopharmacology. 2016;**26**:797-799. DOI: 10.1016/j.euroneuro.2016.04.001

[62] Lloyd EC, Frampton I, Verplanken B, Haase AM. How extreme dieting becomes compulsive: A novel hypothesis for the role of anxiety in the development and maintenance of anorexia nervosa. Medical Hypotheses. 2017;**108**:144-150. DOI: 10.1016/j.mehy.2017.09.001

[63] Kaye WH, Fudge JL, Paulus M. New insights into symptoms and neurocircuit function of anorexia nervosa. Nature Review Neuroscience. 2009;**10**:573-584. DOI: 10.1038/nrn2682

[64] Nunn K, Frampton I, Lask B. Anorexia nervosa—A noradrenergic dysregulation hypothesis. Medical Hypotheses. 2012;**78**:580-584. DOI: 10.1016/j.mehy.2012.01.033

[65] Calati R, De Ronchi D, Bellini M, Serretti A. The 5-HTTLPR polymorphism and eating disorders: A meta-analysis. International Journal of Eating Disorders. 2011;**44**:191-199. DOI: 10.1002/eat.20811

[66] Godier LR, Park RJ. Compulsivity in anorexia nervosa: A transdiagnostic concept. Frontiers in Psychology. 2014;**5**:778. DOI: 10.3389/fpsyg.2014.00778

[67] Figee M, Vink M, de Geus F, Vulink N, Veltman DJ, Westenberg H, et al. Dysfunctional reward circuitry in obsessive-compulsive disorder. Biological Psychiatry. 2011;**69**:867-874. DOI: 10.1016/j.biopsych.2010.12.003

[68] Fontenelle LF, Oostermeijer S, Harrison BJ, Pantelis C, Yücel M. Obsessive-compulsive disorder, impulse control disorders and drug addiction: Common features and potential treatments. Drugs. 2011;**71**:827-840. DOI: 10.2165/11591790-000000000-00000

[69] Chamberlain SR, Lochner C, Stein DJ, Goudriaan AE, van Holst RJ, Zohar J, et al. Behavioural addiction—A rising tide? European Neuropsychopharmacology. 2016;**26**:841-855. DOI: 10.1016/j.euroneuro.2015.08.013

[70] Hart M, Wilcken B, Williams LT, Sibbritt D, Nunn KP. Tyrosine supplementation as an adjunct treatment in anorexia nervosa—A

noradrenergic repletion hypothesis. Advanced Eating Disorder. 2013;**1**:161-168

[71] Haleem DJ. Serotonin neurotransmission in anorexia nervosa. Behavioural Pharmacology. 2012;**23**:478-495. DOI: 10.1097/FBP.0b013e328357440d

[72] Atkinson MJ, Wade TD. Mindfulness-based prevention for eating disorders: A school-based cluster randomized controlled study. International Journal of Eating Disorders. 2015;**48**:1024:37. DOI: 10.1002/eat.22416

[73] Spindler A, Milos G. Links between eating disorder symptom severity and psychiatric comorbidity. Eating Behaviors. 2007;**8**:364-373. DOI: 10.1016/j.eatbeh.2006.11.012

[74] Sternheim L, Startup H, Schmidt U. Anxiety-related processes in anorexia nervosa and their relation to eating disorder pathology, depression and anxiety. Advanced Eating Disorders. 2015;**3**:13-19

[75] Haynos AF, Crosby RD, Engel SG, Lavender JM, Wonderlich SA, Mitchell JE, et al. Initial test of an emotional avoidance model of restriction in anorexia nervosa using ecological momentary assessment. Journal of Psychiatric Research. 2015;**68**:134-139. DOI: 10.1016/j.jpsychires.2015.06.016

[76] Steinglass JE, Sysko R, Mayer L, Berner LA, Schebendach J, Wang Y, et al. Pre-meal anxiety and food intake in anorexia nervosa. Appetite. 2010;**55**:214-218. DOI: 10.1016/j.appet.2010.05.090

[77] Cardi V, Leppanen J, Treasure J. The effects of negative and positive mood induction on eating behaviour: A meta-analysis of laboratory studies in the healthy population and eating and weight disorders. Neuroscience and Biobehavioral Reviews. 2015;**57**:299-309. DOI: 10.1016/j.neubiorev.2015.08.011

[78] Lavender JM, De Young KP, Wonderlich SA, Crosby RD, Engel SG, Mitchell JE, et al. Daily patterns of anxiety in anorexia nervosa: Associations with eating disorder behaviors in the natural environment. Journal of Abnormal Psychology. 2013;**122**:672-683. DOI: 10.1037/a0031823

[79] Gazendam FJ, Kamphuis JH, Kindt M. Deficient safety learning characterizes high trait anxious individuals. Biological Psychology. 2013;**92**:342-352. DOI: 10.1016/j.biopsycho.2012.11.006

[80] Licinio J, Wong ML, Gold PW. The hypothalamic-pituitary-adrenal axis in anorexia nervosa. Psychiatry Research. 1996;**62**:75-83. DOI: 10.1016/0165-1781(96)02991-5

[81] Walsh BT, Roose SP, Katz JL, Dyrenfurth I, Wright L, Vande Wiele R, et al. Hypothalamic-pituitary-adrenal-cortical activity in anorexia nervosa and bulimia. Psychoneuroendocrinology. 1987;**12**:131-140

[82] Fichter MM, Doerr P, Pirke KM, Lund R. Behavior, attitude, nutrition and endocrinology in anorexia nervosa. Acta Psychiatrica Scandinavica. 1982;**66**:429-444. DOI: 10.1111/j.1600-0447.1982.tb04500.x

[83] Jászberényi M, Bujdosó E, Pataki I, Telegdy G. Effect of orexins on the hypothalamic-pituitary-adrenal system. Journal of Neuroendocrinology. 2000;**12**:1174-1178

[84] Griffond B, Risold PY, Jacquemard C, Colard C, Fellmann D. Insulin-induced hypoglycemia increases preprohypocretin (orexin) mRNA in the rat lateral hypothalamic area. Neuroscience Letters. 1999;**262**:77-80. DOI: 10.1016/S0304-3940(98)00976-8

[85] Sakurai T, Amemiya A, Ishii M, Matsuzaki I, Chemelli RM, Tanaka H, et al. Orexins and orexin receptors: A family of hypothalamic neuropéptidos and G protein-coupled receptors that regulate feeding behavior. Cell. 1998;**92**:573-585. DOI: 10.1016/S0092-8674(02)09256-5

[86] Berthoud HR, Munzberg H. The lateral hypothalamus as integrator of metabolic and environmental needs: From electrical self-stimulation to opto-genetics. Physiology & Behavior. 2011;**104**:29-39. DOI: 10.1016/j.physbeh.2011.04.051

[87] Burdakov D, Karnani MM, Gonzalez A. Lateral hypothalamus as a sensor-regulator in respiratory and metabolic control. Physiology & Behavior. 2013;**121**:117-124. DOI: 10.1016/j.physbeh.2013.03.023

[88] Cason AM, Smith RJ, Tahsili-Fahadan P, Moorman DE, Sartor GC, Aston-Jones G. Role of orexin/hypocretin in reward-seeking and addiction: Implications for obesity. Physiology & Behavior. 2010;**100**:419-428. DOI: 10.1016/j.physbeh.2010.03.009

[89] Sheng Z, Santiago AM, Thomas MP, Routh VH. Metabolic regulation of lateral hypothalamic glucose-inhibited orexin neurons may influence midbrain reward neurocircuitry. Molecular and Cellular Neuroscience. 2014;**62**:30-41. DOI: 10.1016/j.mcn.2014.08.001

[90] Yeoh JW, Campbell EJ, James MH, Graham BA, Dayas CV. Orexin antagonists for neuropsychiatric disease: Progress and potential pitfalls. Frontiers in Neuroscience. 2014;**8**:36. DOI: 10.3389/fnins.2014.00036

[91] Salamone JD, Cousins MS, Snyder BJ. Behavioral functions of nucleus accumbens dopamine: Empirical and conceptual problems with the anhedonia hypothesis. Neuroscience and Biobehavioural Review. 1997;**21**:341-359. DOI: 10.1016/S0149-7634(96)00017-6

[92] Cousins MS, Salamone JD. Nucleus accumbens dopamine depletions in rats affect relative response allocation in a novel cost/benefit procedure. Pharmacology Biochemistry and Behavior. 1994;**49**:85-91. DOI: 10.1016/0091-3057(94)90460-X

[93] Nowend KL, Arizzi M, Carlson BB, Salamone JD. D1 or D2 antagonism in nucleus accumbens core or dorsomedial shell suppresses lever pressing for food but leads to compensatory increases in chow consumption. Pharmacology Biochemistry and Behavior. 2001;**69**:373-382. DOI: 10.1016/S0091-3057(01)00524-X

[94] Salamone JD, Arizzi MN, Sandoval MD, Cervone KM, Aberman JE. Dopamine antagonists alter response allocation but do not suppress appetite for food in rats: Contrast between the effects of SKF 83566, raclopride, and fenfluramine on a concurrent choice task. Psychopharmacology. 2002;**160**:371-380. DOI: 10.1007/s00213-001-0994-x

[95] Salamone JD, Steinpreis RE, McCullough LD, Smith P, Grebel D, Mahan K. Haloperidol and nucleus accumbens dopamine depletion suppress lever pressing for food but increase free food consumption in a novel food choice procedure. Psychopharmacology. 1991;**104**:515-521

[96] Ida T, Nakahara K, Murakami T, Hanada R, Nakazato M, Murakami N. Possible involvement of orexin in the stress reaction in rats. Biochemical and Biophysical Research Communications. 2000;**270**:318-323. DOI: 10.1006/bbrc.2000.2412

[97] Abercrombie ED, Keefe KA, DiFrischia DS, Zigmond MJ. Differential effect of stress on in vivo dopamine

release in striatum, nucleus accumbens, and medial frontal cortex. Journal of Neurochemistry. 1989;**52**:1655-1658. DOI: 10.1111/j.1471-4159.1989.tb09224.x

[98] Imperato A, Angelucci L, Casoloni P, Zocchi A, Puglisi-Allegra S. Repeated stressful experiences differently affect limbic dopamine release during and following stress. Brain Research. 1992;**577**:194-199. DOI: 10.1016/0006-8993(92)90274-D

[99] Pezze MA, Feldon J. Mesolimbic dopaminergic pathways in fear conditioning. Progress in Neurobiology. 2004;**74**:301-320. DOI: 10.1016/j.pneurobio.2004.09.004

[100] Sim H, Choi T-Y, Lee HJ, Kang EY, Yoon S, Han P-L, et al. Role of dopamine D2 receptors in plasticity of stress-induced addictive behaviours. Nature Communications. 2013;**4**:1579-1589. DOI: 10.1038/ncomms2598

[101] Cabib S, Giardino L, Calzá L, Zanni M, Mele A, Puglisi-Allegra S. Stress promotes major changes in dopamine densities within the mesoaccumbens and nigrostriatal systems. Neuroscience. 1998;**84**:193-200. DOI: 10.1016/S0306-4522(97)00468-5

Chapter 6

Dysbiosis of the Microbiota in Anorexia Nervosa: Pathophysiological Implications

Magnus Sjögren, Stein Frostad and Kenneth Klingenberg Barfod

Abstract

Anorexia nervosa (AN) is a severe and often enduring condition of which the etiology is unknown. Studies on the gut microbiota in AN have found deviations from that of healthy individuals, which may imply a relation to pathophysiology, development and maintenance of the disorder via the gut-brain axis, which has been shown in other disorders. A narrative review of the gut microbiota studies in AN is presented. Several studies point to a dysbiosis in AN which may have implications for maintenance of a low body weight, immunological changes and a severely reduced food intake. An association may be found to clinical symptoms in AN. A pathophysiological model for disease is presented implying a role of the microbiota in maintenance of AN. Dysbiosis in AN may play an important role in the development and maintenance of AN.

Keywords: anorexia nervosa, feces, microbiota, species, biomarkers

1. Introduction

Anorexia nervosa (AN) is a serious and often enduring psychiatric condition. The hallmark features of AN are a phobia for weight gain, and for intake of fattening food, disturbance in body image, and often compensatory behaviors such as excessive exercise and purging, which overall leads to a reduction of energy intake relative to energy expenditure leading to low body weight. An increased risk of suicide and frequent potential life-threatening medical complications of several body organs contribute to AN having a high standardized mortality ratio of 5.2 [3.7–7.5] [1]. This is coupled with a high risk of enduring disease [2].

The weight loss is in some patients preceded by a depression, a trauma, gastrointestinal symptoms or an infection. But in a majority of patients there is no detectable psychiatric or somatic disorder preceding the weight loss. In children and adolescents with AN, family-based treatment as described by Lock and LeGrange is recommended [3] and if treatment is started shortly after debut of the disorder, the prognosis is fairly good. However, if treatment is delayed, the prognosis becomes worse [4]. In adults, individual eating-disorder-focused therapy (CBT-ED) is recommended [5]. With this treatment, drop-out rates are high and even with optimal treatment by well-trained therapists only 50% of the patients who start CBT-ED have good effect of the therapy [6, 7].

Considering the high mortality, high chronicity and lack of knowledge on the etiology of AN, there is an immense need for an improved understanding of the etiology and pathophysiology of the disease in order to find ways to better treatments. This knowledge would preferably explain both the routes into developing the disorder and mechanisms that serve to maintain it, and proposedly involve both biological and psychological factors, such that measures and biomarkers to follow the development and recovery from of the disease could be identified. Potential further benefits with biomarkers for AN may be guidance for risk stratification, treatment and target identification for novel treatments. The last few years have seen an increase in studies on the gut microbiota and its associated microbiome which might harbor trait biomarkers for AN.

The "microbiota" refers to the cumulative microorganisms, including Bacteria, Viruses, Archaea, Protists and Fungi, which populate a number of human tissues and biofluids including the skin, lungs, roal mucosa, saliva, and gastrointestinal tract, and the "microbiome" refers to the collective genomes of the present microorganisms [8]. There are more than 1000 'species-level' phylotypes that coexist in a human [9], and the majority of these phylotypes are Bacteria, with *Faecalibacterium prausnitzii*, *Roseburia intestinalis*, and *Bacteroides uniformis* dominating in the adult microbiota found in feces samples [10]. The composition of the phylotypes is mostly consistent across individuals, albeit there may be a large variability with regard to relative composition and diversity of the included microorganisms, intra-individually depending on anatomical site and inter-individually at the same anatomical location. In addition, there are inter-individual variations at the same anatomical site.

The gut microbiota is critical for the development of the gut mucosal immunity [11, 12], and it is also involved in the regulation of the hypothalamic-pituitary-adrenal (HPA) axis [13], serotonergic neurotransmission [14], and signaling mechanisms affecting neuronal circuits involved in motor control and anxiety in mice [15]. This pathway has been named the gut-brain axis [16].

2. The gut-brain axis

The existence of the gut-brain axis is exemplified by irritable bowel syndrome (IBS) where more than half of the patients also suffer from mood disorders and for which antidepressants is one of the more common pharmaceutical treatments [17]. In IBS and other potential gut-brain axis disorders, cognitive alterations seem to be key features of the disorders [18]. These cognitive alterations might be induced by signal transduction from gut to the brain [18]. In addition, the existence is also shown by the effects of antibiotic exposure, which may lead to altered brain function such as anxiety, panic disorder, major depression, psychosis, and delirium which are usually described as side effects of antibiotic treatment [19]. Support for the latter comes also from studies in mice which have shown that an altered composition of the gut microbiota in adult mice, and an increased exploratory behavioral including hippocampal expression of Brain Derived Nerve growth Factor (BDNF) has been found after oral administration of non-absorbable antimicrobials [20], in contrast to intraperitoneal administration, which had no effect on behavior or BDNF levels.

Another area of evidence for the gut-brain-axis stems from dietary induction of changes in gut microbiota and linked psychopathological outcomes. For example, a high fat diet has been found associated with an altered microbial diversity and diminished synaptic plasticity [21, 22] but also increased vulnerability and anxiety-like behavior in the mice [23]. In addition, a diet high in sucrose also led to an altered microbial diversity associated with impaired development of spatial bias for long term memory, short term memory, and reversal trainings [24]. Another strong evidence for the gut-brain axis comes from a study in mice exposed to a microbiome depletion and/or transplantation paradigm where microbiota, in a first step, was isolated from donors who were provided with either in high fat diet or a controlled diet, and thereafter in a second step, transfused to mice who developed significant and selective disruptions in exploratory, cognitive, and also developed the stereotypical behavior following the high fat diet [25]. However, there are also evidence from studies where alcohol exposure, smoking habits, and disruptions in diurnal rhythm all have been shown to affect the microbiota composition.

There are also other evidence pointing to a reciprocal interaction from a study where a second generation antipsychotics, olanzapine, was exposed to rats and found to affect the composition of the microbiota, which also triggered an inflammatory response and weight gain [26, 27]. Furthermore, the exposure to antibiotics seemed to attenuate these physiological effects [28].

The microbiome has also been found to have been altered in various psychiatric conditions, or to affect its clinical expression, as well altered in rodent models for these disorders [29]. One example is major depressive disorder (MDD) where, for example, in germ-free mice (mice completely void of bacterial microbiota or derived molecules), there are both changes from comparable normal mice in the hypothalamic, pituitary, adrenal stress response, as well as altered levels of monoamines concentrations or their receptors [13–15, 20, 30]. Indirect evidence in MDD also comes from an increased serum antibody level to lipopolysaccharides that stems from Gram-negative enterobacteria, which are higher in MDD compared to controls [31], and which is associated with stress associated increased gut permeability and bacterial translocation in animal models [32, 33]. In addition, depression also altered the gut microbiota in a mouse model, in which chronic depression and anxiety-like behaviors were induced by olfactory bulbectomy [34], suggesting a feedback loop between depressive states and dysbiosis.

Furthermore, a similar type of relation between dysbiosis and psychopathogenesis is found in schizophrenia [35, 36]. For example, elevated levels of serological markers of bacterial translocation have been found to be highly correlated with systemic inflammatory markers in schizophrenia [37], and, cytokine levels in schizophrenia are correlated with the severity of symptomatology [38]. From a genetic point of view, several of the strongest associations identified between genetic risk and schizophrenia stems from genes that are linked to immunological function [57, 58]. This is particularly interesting in view of the genetic association between AN and schizophrenia [39].

3. How is the effects in the gut-brain axis mediated?

The mechanism behind the gut brain axis may be multifaceted involving neural signal transduction in nervus vagus, neurotransmitters, immunological mechanisms, and mechanisms related to metabolism and energy utilization [40]. One of the strongest links from a mechanistic point of view, stems from research on serotonin and the microbiota. Enterochromaffin (EC) cells provides approximately 95% of the total body content of serotonin [41] of which the majority exists in plasma. Multiple levels of evidence links disturbances in the serotonergic system and several psychiatric disorder such as depression, anxiety, and borderline personality disorder. For example, the metabolism of tryptophan, a precursor of serotonin, is potentially regulated by the gut microbiota thereby enabling it to influence brain function [42]. Tryptophan is an essential amino acid derived from the diet [43], and tryptophan that is absorbed from the gut into the bloodstream passes the blood-brain barrier to contribute to serotonin synthesis in situ [43]. The availability of tryptophan is strongly affected by the gut microbiota, and several studies have indicated that bacteria such as streptococcus, Escherichia, enterococcus species and *Bifidobacterium infantis*, and especially indigenous spore-forming bacteria may modulate serotonin levels by increasing plasma tryptophan [44]. An example of this is studies in germ free mice that have found that they exhibit an increased plasma tryptophan concentration [14, 15], which after post weaning colonization can be normalized [14]. The serotonergic neurotransmission may thereby be influenced by the availability of tryptophan for serotonin production [45]. There are studies have found that a depletion of tryptophan influences mood, anxiety and borderline personality traits, for example, in AN and bulimia nervosa [46–49].

There are also other evidences that link the gut microbiota with psychiatric conditions such as MDD. For examples, a recent publication by Seng et al. [50] provides three additional levels of evidences: (a) that germ free mice lacks gut microbiota and display depression like features in forced swimming test compared to conventionally raised healthy control mice; (b) that the gut microbiota composition of MDD patients differ from that of healthy controls; and (c) and that transplantation of MDD microbiota to germ free mice led to the development of depression like behaviors. In addition, Seng et al. found that mice that were harboring the microbiota from MDD patients primarily exhibited disturbances of microbiome genes and host metabolism which thereby suggests that the depression-like behavior was mediated through the host metabolism [50].

Another neurotransmitter that is produced by the microbiota and that may influence host behavior is gamma aminobutyric acid (GABA) which is the main inhibitory neurotransmitter in the CNS. GABA produced by the probiotic *Lactobacillus rhamnosus* was administered to mice and led to an alteration in the expression of GABA receptors in different CNS regions, associated with reduced anxiety and depression-like behaviors [51].

Another mechanism for interaction between the microbiome and the CNS is at the level of the blood-brain barrier (BBB). The vascular BBB is comprised of specialized brain endothelial cells acts as a regulatory interface between brain and blood that prevent the unrestricted transfer of molecules into the CNS. Disruption of the tight junctions of the BBB can expose the CNS, and has also been linked to CNS disorders [52]. A dysbiotic microbiome could possibly interact with the BBB in several ways: bacterial factors and immune-active molecules released from peripheral sites influenced by the microbiome can cross the BBB, alter BBB integrity or change BBB transport [53]. In germ-free mice, it has been shown that the BBB has increased permeability compared to pathogen-free mice with a normal gut flora. The increased permeability was associated with reduced expression of the tight junction proteins. Exposure of germ-free adult mice to a normal gut microbiota decreased BBB permeability and up-regulated the expression of tight junction proteins [54]. Metabolic products such as short-chain fatty acids (SCFAs) are produced through the fermentation of dietary fibers by the gut microbiota [55] and can cross the BBB to affect brain function. A low production of SCFAs could lead to increased BBB permeability and SCFAs has been shown to be able to improve a dysfunctional BBB in germ-free mice [54]. Another example is that antibiotics are able to modify barrier integrity and alter behavior in mice [56] and alterations to the microbiome composition in mice in favor of, for example, probiotic bifidobacteria spp. through food supplement with prebiotics showed impact on neuroinflammation and were accompanied with changes in the expression of tight junction proteins [57]. Furthermore, leptin, a key hormone for the control of appetite and weight gain, is normally restricted by the BBB but has been shown in mice with a deficit in leptin transport to the brain to enhance the sense of food reward [58].

4. Microbiota findings in AN studies

Dysbiosis has been proposed in AN and through the long periods of starvation associated with the core psychopathology of AN, a considerable adaptation in gut microbiota could occur in individuals with AN. A systematic review by Schwennsen et al. [59] found some evidence of dysbiosis in AN, such as the abundance of the gut microbiota in AN, which was described as either normal [60, 61], reduced [62] or altered in AN [63]. In addition, the diversity of the gut microbiota in AN was described as normal [61, 63], or reduced (alpha, i.e., within-sample diversity) [64] both in the acute stage and after weight restoration.

Common microbiota findings in the acute stages of AN were low levels of phylum Bacteroidetes [61, 64], while the phylum Firmicutes was increased in AN in three studies [61, 64, 65] however decreased in a fourth [63]. Furthermore, the genus *Methanobrevibacter* and specifically, the species *M. smithii*, has been found increased in AN patients in several studies [60, 61, 63, 65]. It is important to remember the presence or lack of a specific bacterial spp. identified by their 16rRNA gene is not the same as the presences or lack of certain metabolic functions or microbiota steady-state dynamic. The state of knowledge of the microbiota in AN is in its infancy and more studies are needed.

4.1 The microbiota and relation to clinical symptoms in AN

This systematic review [59] identified two studies describing an association between the microbiota and clinical symptoms in AN. In one study, ClpB protein concentrations were significantly correlated with several subscales on the Eating Disorder Inventory-2 (EDI-2) for patients with eating disorders and the Montgomery-Åsberg Depression Rating Scale (MADRS) total score and specifically the anhedonia score for AN patients ($p < 0.05$) [66]. In another study, an association between alpha diversity and depression and eating disorder psychopathology was found in AN [64]. Should further studies find further support for that the microbiota drives the symptoms of AN, this would strengthen targeting the microbiota as a primary level of treatment of AN.

5. How is the gut-brain axis involved in AN? Breakdown of organic material in the gut and its exposure in plasma

A potential mechanism through which the microbiota indirectly influences the pathophysiology and symptoms of AN is through the breakdown of organic material in the gut and the transfer of metabolites into the blood stream. One of the microbiota that has been described in AN is *M. smithii,* which is involved in the breakdown of polysaccharides from vegetable sources and the finding of this specific Archaeon could illustrate an adaptation to a typical diet rich in vegetables and fruits in persons with AN. In addition, methanogenic Archaea, such as *M. smithii*, have also been linked to constipation, a common complaint in patients with AN, which statins have been shown to alleviate by suppressing the growth of methanogens [65, 67–69]. The evidence of *M. smithii* in feces from constipated patients necessitate further investigation of whether this finding in AN patients is only related to constipation or also related to AN psychopathology as a potential biomarker.

The gut microbiota is involved in both weight gain and weight loss as well as with energy extraction from the diet in both humans and animals [70, 71]. Differences in the composition of the gut microbiota between obese and lean individuals have been consistently described, potentially illustrating differences in energy extraction efficiency between obese and lean individuals [72, 73], and specific gut dysbiosis could predispose to the drive toward negative energy balance in AN. With regard to the effect of weight gain on the fecal microbiota, Firmicutes has been found increased after weight restoration in two studies in AN [61, 64].

6. AN comorbid disorder as evidence of microbiota influence

Intestinal dysbiosis has previously been associated with psychological function and mental health including depression and anxiety, both of which are commonly comorbid with AN [40]. AN patients often present with comorbid anxiety (75% lifetime prevalence of anxiety disorder) [74] and depression (more than 34% lifetime prevalence of depression) [75, 76]. These findings provide further support for a role of dysbiosis in the pathophysiology of AN.

7. A leaking gut in AN?

During starvation, some of the gut bacteria will have insufficient nutrient supply for survival. Slowly growing bacteria or bacteria able to feed on the mucus lining the gut wall will survive for a longer period of time [77]. The competition between bacteria with different growth capacities to survive and proliferate in the gut has probably taken place for millions of years. Thus, it is reasonable to expect that various mechanisms for survival and proliferation have emerged among gut bacteria including the capacity to release of substances inhibiting food intake of the host. Alterations in gut permeability has been linked to a number of intestinal diseases, such as irritable bowel syndrome (IBS), inflammatory bowel disease (IBD), but also to extraintestinal disease as depression, anxiety and autism specter disorders [78, 79]. Increased gut permeability may also facilitate signal transduction from the gut to the brain via the vagus nerve and blood [80], possibly in synergy with interaction with increased BBB permeability. In addition, in animal and human studies, the experience of stress is also linked to an increase in permeability of the intestinal barrier. This increase in permeability seems to be mediated through, among other factors, hypothalamic hormones, especially corticotropi-releasing hormone (CRH) [77]. Increased mucin degrading bacteria has been demonstrated in AN [81] indicating that decreased food intake induce overgrowth of bacteria able to feed on the mucus layer and thereby increase gut permeability.

An example of a possible biomarker species is the bacterium *Akkermansia muciniphila* which is abundant in humans and rodents and has been inversely correlates with body weight and is associated with metabolic syndromes and auto-immune diseases [82]. *A. municiphilia* is a symbiotic bacterium of the mucus layer, can utilize mucin as its sole carbon, nitrogen, and energy source and is able to produce certain SCFAs [83, 84]. In mice, it has been shown that the abundance of *A. muciniphila* decreased in obese and type 2 diabetic mice and that administration of the bacterium increased the intestinal levels of endocannabinoids that control inflammation, the gut barrier, and gut peptide secretion [82]. In a single AN patient case story, it has been shown that one treatment with a fecal matter transplant from a healthy donor led to weight gain and an increase in *A. municiphilia* and SCFAs blood levels [85]. *A. municiphilia* is an example of a complex interaction where the bacterium simultaneously degrade the mucin for energy, but also at the same time induces higher mucus production from the host. This could in turn improve protection of the gut wall from interaction with harmful molecules from other gut bacteria and leakage into the blood.

Furthermore, in an activity based mouse model of AN Jésus et al. demonstrated increased permeability in the colon, that is, "gut leakiness", in anorexic mice, however the authors also found that the gut leakiness was more related to malnutrition than exercise [86]. Although there may be conflicting studies [87], yet another study examining the role of exercise on gut permeability, found that exercise increases intestinal permeability measured with the lactulose and rhamnose differential urinary excretion test [88].

Another support for a leaking gut wall in AN comes from a study by Breton et al. [66], who found an increase in ClpB protein concentrations in plasma in eating disorder patients compared to plasma of controls, and furthermore, that ClpB protein concentrations correlated positively with alpha-Melanocyte Stimulating Hormone-(alpha-MSH)-reactive IgG for all patients with eating disorders. ClpB protein is produced by *Enterobacteriae* such as *Escherichia coli* and has been found as a conformational mimetic of alpha-MSH, which is thought to be involved in satiety and anxiety [89]. The study adds evidence to the potential role of ClpB protein produced by *Enterobacteriae* in the gut and its impact on the brain and psychopathology in eating disorders.

The potentially altered gut permeability in AN may underlie the low-grade inflammation and increased risk of autoimmune diseases found in eating disorders [90]. Moreover, starvation has a significant impact on the gut microbiota, and a diet based on animal products used for re-nutrition, may stimulate the growth of bacteria that trigger inflammation [91].

8. A model for the pathophysiology of AN

The initial reduction of food intake induces alterations in the gut microbiota. These alterations in gut microbiota induce increased gut permeability. Due to this

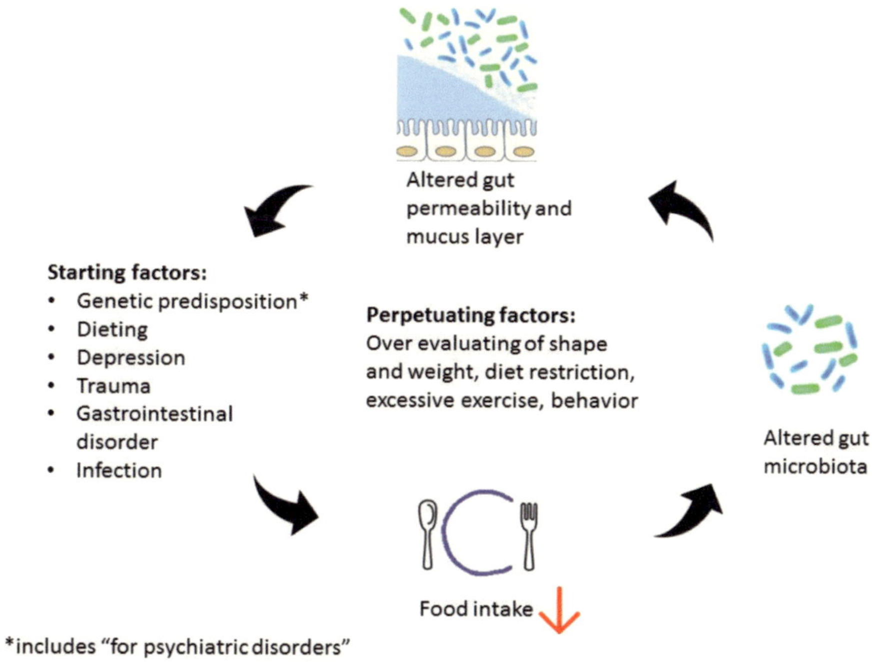

Figure 1.
The initial reduction of food intake induces alterations in the gut microbiota. These alterations in gut microbiota induce increased gut permeability. Due to this altered microbiota and increased gut and in addition, increased blood-brain barrier permeability, neurohormonal signals interfering with food intake are transferred to the brain, influencing brain functions, for example, cognition. This contributes in creating a vicious circle which subserves maintaining in the mechanisms associated with AN.

altered microbiota and increased gut and in addition, increased blood-brain barrier permeability, neurohormonal signals interfering with food intake are transferred to the brain, influencing brain functions, for example, cognition. This contributes in creating a vicious circle which subserves in maintaining the mechanisms associated with AN (**Figure 1**).

9. Conclusions

There are a lot of evidence linking dysbiosis and inflammatory and psychiatric disorders and although there are only a few studies that have examined the microbiota in AN, several of these point to a dysbiosis also in AN. The effects of this dysbiosis is mediated through the gut-brain axis, and leakage through the gut and potentially also the BBB, provide pathways for neurohormonal signals to induce and maintain psychiatric disorders such as AN. The evidence in AN will need confirmation and further clarification in larger, randomized and controlled studies. We propose a model for disease development and maintenance in AN where a dysbiosis is a key component. Future studies will need to clarify the pathophysiology of AN.

Acknowledgements

We are thankful to Psychiatric Center Ballerup and the Capitol Region of Denmark, for providing support for this study.

Conflict of interest

The authors declare no conflict of interest.

Author details

Magnus Sjögren[1,2*], Stein Frostad[3] and Kenneth Klingenberg Barfod[4]

1 Mental Health Center Ballerup, Ballerup, Denmark

2 Institute for Clinical Medicine, University of Copenhagen, Denmark

3 Department of Mental Health Research, Division of Psychiatry, Haukeland University Hospital, Bergen, Norway

4 Department of Veterinary and Animal Sciences, Section of Experimental Animal Models, University of Copenhagen, Denmark

*Address all correspondence to: jan.magnus.sjoegren@regionh.dk

References

[1] Keshaviah A et al. Re-examining premature mortality in anorexia nervosa: A meta-analysis redux. Comprehensive Psychiatry. 2014;**55**(8):1773-1784

[2] Steinhausen HC. Outcome of eating disorders. Child and Adolescent Psychiatric Clinics of North America. 2009;**18**(1):225-242

[3] Lock J, Le Grange D. Treatment Manual for Anorexia Nervosa: A Family-Based Approach. 2nd ed. New York; London: Guilford; 2013

[4] Treasure J, Russell G. The case for early intervention in anorexia nervosa: Theoretical exploration of maintaining factors. The British Journal of Psychiatry. 2011;**199**(1):5-7

[5] Eating Disorders: Recognition and treatment. Clinical Guideline, National Guideline Alliance (UK). London: National Institute for Health and Care Excellence; 2017. https://www.nice.org.uk/guidance/NG69 [Accessed 1 Mar 2019]

[6] Cooper Z, Fairburn CG. The evolution of "enhanced" cognitive behavior therapy for eating disorders: Learning from treatment nonresponse. Cognitive and Behavioral Practice. 2011;**18**(3):394-402

[7] Frostad S et al. Implementation of enhanced cognitive behaviour therapy (CBT-E) for adults with anorexia nervosa in an outpatient eating-disorder unit at a public hospital. Journal of Eating Disorders. 2018;**6**:12

[8] Quigley EMM. Gut bacteria in health and disease. Gastroenterology & Hepatology. 2013;**9**(9):560-569

[9] Claesson MJ et al. Comparative analysis of pyrosequencing and a phylogenetic microarray for exploring microbial community structures in the human distal intestine. PLoS One. 2009;**4**(8):e6669

[10] Qin J et al. A human gut microbial gene catalogue established by metagenomic sequencing. Nature. 2010;**464**(7285):59-65

[11] Sudo N et al. The requirement of intestinal bacterial flora for the development of an IgE production system fully susceptible to oral tolerance induction. Journal of Immunology. 1997;**159**(4):1739-1745

[12] Guarner F, Malagelada JR. Gut flora in health and disease. Lancet. 2003;**361**(9356):512-519

[13] Sudo N et al. Postnatal microbial colonization programs the hypothalamic-pituitary-adrenal system for stress response in mice. The Journal of Physiology. 2004;**558**(Pt 1): 263-275

[14] Clarke G et al. The microbiome-gut-brain axis during early life regulates the hippocampal serotonergic system in a sex-dependent manner. Molecular Psychiatry. 2013;**18**(6):666-673

[15] Diaz Heijtz R et al. Normal gut microbiota modulates brain development and behavior. Proceedings of the National Academy of Sciences of the United States of America. 2011;**108**(7):3047-3052

[16] Cryan JF, O'Mahony SM. The microbiome-gut-brain axis: From bowel to behavior. Neurogastroenterology and Motility. 2011;**23**(3):187-192

[17] Neufeld KA, Foster JA. Effects of gut microbiota on the brain: Implications for psychiatry. Journal of Psychiatry & Neuroscience. 2009;**34**(3):230-231

[18] Kennedy PJ et al. Irritable bowel syndrome: A microbiome-gut-brain axis disorder? World Journal of Gastroenterology. 2014;**20**(39):14105-14125

[19] Sternbach H, State R. Antibiotics: Neuropsychiatric effects and psychotropic interactions. Harvard Review of Psychiatry. 1997;**5**(4):214-226

[20] Bercik P et al. The intestinal microbiota affect central levels of brain-derived neurotropic factor and behavior in mice. Gastroenterology. 2011;**141**(2):599-609, 609 e1-3

[21] Liu Z et al. High-fat diet induces hepatic insulin resistance and impairment of synaptic plasticity. PLoS One. 2015;**10**(5):e0128274

[22] Daniel H et al. High-fat diet alters gut microbiota physiology in mice. The ISME Journal. 2014;**8**(2):295-308

[23] Sharma S, Fernandes MF, Fulton S. Adaptations in brain reward circuitry underlie palatable food cravings and anxiety induced by high-fat diet withdrawal. International Journal of Obesity. 2013;**37**(9):1183-1191

[24] Magnusson KR et al. Relationships between diet-related changes in the gut microbiome and cognitive flexibility. Neuroscience. 2015;**300**:128-140

[25] Bruce-Keller AJ et al. Obese-type gut microbiota induce neurobehavioral changes in the absence of obesity. Biological Psychiatry. 2015;**77**(7):607-615

[26] Davey KJ et al. Gender-dependent consequences of chronic olanzapine in the rat: Effects on body weight, inflammatory, metabolic and microbiota parameters. Psychopharmacology. 2012;**221**(1):155-169

[27] Ley RE et al. Microbial ecology: Human gut microbes associated with obesity. Nature. 2006;**444**(7122):1022-1023

[28] Davey KJ et al. Antipsychotics and the gut microbiome: Olanzapine-induced metabolic dysfunction is attenuated by antibiotic administration in the rat. Translational Psychiatry. 2013;**3**:e309

[29] Hansen AK et al. A review of applied aspects of dealing with gut microbiota impact on rodent models. ILAR Journal. 2015;**56**(2):250-264

[30] Neufeld KM et al. Reduced anxiety-like behavior and central neurochemical change in germ-free mice. Neurogastroenterology and Motility. 2011;**23**(3):255-264, e119

[31] Maes M, Kubera M, Leunis JC. The gut-brain barrier in major depression: Intestinal mucosal dysfunction with an increased translocation of LPS from gram negative enterobacteria (leaky gut) plays a role in the inflammatory pathophysiology of depression. Neuro Endocrinology Letters. 2008;**29**(1):117-124

[32] Bravo JA et al. Communication between gastrointestinal bacteria and the nervous system. Current Opinion in Pharmacology. 2012;**12**(6):667-672

[33] Ait-Belgnaoui A et al. Acute stress-induced hypersensitivity to colonic distension depends upon increase in paracellular permeability: Role of myosin light chain kinase. Pain. 2005;**113**(1-2):141-147

[34] Park AJ et al. Altered colonic function and microbiota profile in a mouse model of chronic depression. Neurogastroenterology and Motility. 2013;**25**(9):733-e575

[35] Dinan TG, Borre YE, Cryan JF. Genomics of schizophrenia: Time to consider the gut microbiome? Molecular Psychiatry. 2014;**19**(12):1252-1257

[36] Nemani K et al. Schizophrenia and the gut-brain axis. Progress in Neuro-Psychopharmacology & Biological Psychiatry. 2015;**56**:155-160

[37] Severance EG et al. Discordant patterns of bacterial translocation markers and implications for innate immune imbalances in schizophrenia. Schizophrenia Research. 2013;**148**(1-3):130-137

[38] Fan X, Goff DC, Henderson DC. Inflammation and schizophrenia. Expert Review of Neurotherapeutics. 2007;**7**(7):789-796

[39] Duncan L et al. Significant locus and metabolic genetic correlations revealed in genome-wide association study of anorexia nervosa. The American Journal of Psychiatry. 2017;**174**(9):850-858

[40] Rogers GB et al. From gut dysbiosis to altered brain function and mental illness: Mechanisms and pathways. Molecular Psychiatry. 2016;**21**(6):738-748

[41] Erspamer V. Pharmacology of indole-alkylamines. Pharmacological Reviews. 1954;**6**(4):425-487

[42] O'Mahony SM et al. Serotonin, tryptophan metabolism and the brain-gut-microbiome axis. Behavioural Brain Research. 2015;**277**:32-48

[43] Ruddick JP et al. Tryptophan metabolism in the central nervous system: Medical implications. Expert Reviews in Molecular Medicine. 2006;**8**(20):1-27

[44] Yano JM et al. Indigenous bacteria from the gut microbiota regulate host serotonin biosynthesis. Cell. 2015;**161**(2):264-276

[45] Ben-Ari Y. Neuropaediatric and neuroarchaeology: Understanding development to correct brain disorders. Acta Paediatrica. 2013;**102**(4):331-334

[46] Kaye WH et al. Anxiolytic effects of acute tryptophan depletion in anorexia nervosa. The International Journal of Eating Disorders. 2003;**33**(3):257-267. Discussion 268-70

[47] Kaye WH et al. Effects of acute tryptophan depletion on mood in bulimia nervosa. Biological Psychiatry. 2000;**47**(2):151-157

[48] Smith KA, Fairburn CG, Cowen PJ. Symptomatic relapse in bulimia nervosa following acute tryptophan depletion. Archives of General Psychiatry. 1999;**56**(2):171-176

[49] Weltzin TE et al. Acute tryptophan depletion and increased food intake and irritability in bulimia nervosa. The American Journal of Psychiatry. 1995;**152**(11):1668-1671

[50] Zheng P et al. Gut microbiome remodeling induces depressive-like behaviors through a pathway mediated by the host's metabolism. Molecular Psychiatry. 2016;**21**(6):786-796

[51] Bravo JA et al. Ingestion of lactobacillus strain regulates emotional behavior and central GABA receptor expression in a mouse via the vagus nerve. Proceedings of the National Academy of Sciences of the United States of America. 2011;**108**(38):16050-16055

[52] Najjar S et al. Neurovascular unit dysfunction and blood-brain barrier hyperpermeability contribute to schizophrenia neurobiology: A theoretical integration of clinical and experimental evidence. Front Psychiatry. 2017;**8**:83

[53] Logsdon AF et al. Gut reactions: How the blood-brain barrier connects the microbiome and the brain. Experimental Biology

and Medicine (Maywood, N.J.). 2018;**243**(2):159-165

[54] Braniste V et al. The gut microbiota influences blood-brain barrier permeability in mice. Science Translational Medicine. 2014;**6**(263):263ra158

[55] Topping DL, Clifton PM. Short-chain fatty acids and human colonic function: Roles of resistant starch and nonstarch polysaccharides. Physiological Reviews. 2001;**81**(3):1031-1064

[56] Leclercq S et al. Low-dose penicillin in early life induces long-term changes in murine gut microbiota, brain cytokines and behavior. Nature Communications. 2017;**8**:15062

[57] de Cossio LF et al. Impact of prebiotics on metabolic and behavioral alterations in a mouse model of metabolic syndrome. Brain, Behavior, and Immunity. 2017;**64**:33-49

[58] Di Spiezio A et al. The LepR-mediated leptin transport across brain barriers controls food reward. Molecuar Metabolism. 2018;**8**:13-22

[59] Schwensen HF et al. A systematic review of studies on the faecal microbiota in anorexia nervosa: Future research may need to include microbiota from the small intestine. Eating and Weight Disorders. 2018;**23**(4):399-418

[60] Million M et al. Correlation between body mass index and gut concentrations of *Lactobacillus reuteri*, Bifidobacterium animalis, *Methanobrevibacter smithii* and *Escherichia coli*. International Journal of Obesity. 2013;**37**(11):1460-1466

[61] Mack I et al. Weight gain in anorexia nervosa does not ameliorate the faecal microbiota, branched chain fatty acid profiles, and gastrointestinal complaints. Scientific Reports. 2016;**6**:26752

[62] Morita C et al. Gut dysbiosis in patients with anorexia nervosa. PLoS One. 2015;**10**(12):e0145274

[63] Borgo F et al. Microbiota in anorexia nervosa: The triangle between bacterial species, metabolites and psychological tests. PLoS One. 2017;**12**(6):e0179739

[64] Kleiman SC et al. The intestinal microbiota in acute anorexia nervosa and during renourishment: Relationship to depression, anxiety, and eating disorder psychopathology. Psychosomatic Medicine. 2015;**77**(9):969-981

[65] Armougom F et al. Monitoring bacterial community of human gut microbiota reveals an increase in lactobacillus in obese patients and methanogens in anorexic patients. PLoS One. 2009;**4**(9):e7125

[66] Breton J et al. Elevated plasma concentrations of bacterial ClpB protein in patients with eating disorders. The International Journal of Eating Disorders. 2016;**49**(8):805-808

[67] Samuel BS, Gordon JI. A humanized gnotobiotic mouse model of host-archaeal-bacterial mutualism. Proceedings of the National Academy of Sciences of the United States of America. 2006;**103**(26):10011-10016

[68] Gottlieb K et al. Review article: Inhibition of methanogenic archaea by statins as a targeted management strategy for constipation and related disorders. Alimentary Pharmacology & Therapeutics. 2016;**43**(2):197-212

[69] Triantafyllou K, Chang C, Pimentel M. Methanogens, methane and gastrointestinal motility. Journal of Neurogastroenterology and Motility. 2014;**20**(1):31-40

[70] Flint HJ. Obesity and the gut microbiota. Journal of

Clinical Gastroenterology. 2011;**45**(Suppl):S128-S132

[71] Cox LM, Blaser MJ. Pathways in microbe-induced obesity. Cell Metabolism. 2013;**17**(6):883-894

[72] Aguirre M et al. In vitro characterization of the impact of different substrates on metabolite production, energy extraction and composition of gut microbiota from lean and obese subjects. PLoS One. 2014;**9**(11):e113864

[73] Turnbaugh PJ et al. A core gut microbiome in obese and lean twins. Nature. 2009;**457**(7228):480-484

[74] Godart NT et al. Anxiety disorders in anorexia nervosa and bulimia nervosa: Co-morbidity and chronology of appearance. European Psychiatry. 2000;**15**(1):38-45

[75] Fernandez-Aranda F et al. Symptom profile of major depressive disorder in women with eating disorders. The Australian and New Zealand Journal of Psychiatry. 2007;**41**(1):24-31

[76] Kask J, Ekselius L, Brandt L, Kollia N, Ekbom A, and Papadopoulos FC. Mortality in women with anorexia nervosa: The role of comorbid psychiatric disorders. Psychosomatic Medicine. 2016;**78**(8):910-919

[77] Herpertz-Dahlmann B, Seitz J, Baines J. Food matters: How the microbiome and gut-brain interaction might impact the development and course of anorexia nervosa. European Child & Adolescent Psychiatry. 2017;**26**(9):1031-1041

[78] Goyette P et al. Molecular pathogenesis of inflammatory bowel disease: Genotypes, phenotypes and personalized medicine. Annals of Medicine. 2007;**39**(3):177-199

[79] Spiller RC. Overlap between irritable bowel syndrome and inflammatory bowel disease. Digestive Diseases. 2009;**27**(Suppl 1): 48-54

[80] Ntranos A, Casaccia P. The microbiome-gut-behavior axis: Crosstalk between the gut microbiome and oligodendrocytes modulates behavioral responses. Neurotherapeutics. 2018;**15**(1):31-35

[81] Mack I et al. Is the impact of starvation on the gut microbiota specific or unspecific to anorexia nervosa? A narrative review based on a systematic literature search. Current Neuropharmacology. 2018;**16**(8):1131-1149

[82] Everard A et al. Cross-talk between *Akkermansia muciniphila* and intestinal epithelium controls diet-induced obesity. Proceedings of the National Academy of Sciences of the United States of America. 2013;**110**(22):9066-9071

[83] Derrien M et al. The Mucin degrader *Akkermansia muciniphila* is an abundant resident of the human intestinal tract. Applied and Environmental Microbiology. 2008;**74**(5):1646-1648

[84] Zhai Q et al. A next generation probiotic, *Akkermansia muciniphila*. Critical Reviews in Food Science and Nutrition. 2018:1-10. https://doi.org/10.1080/10408398.2018.1517725

[85] de Clercq NC, Frissen MN, Davids M, Groen AK, and Nieuwdorp M. Weight gain after fecal microbiota transplantation in a patient with recurrent underweight following clinical recovery from anorexia nervosa. Psychotherapy and Psychosomatics. 2019;**88**:58-60

[86] Jesus P et al. Alteration of intestinal barrier function during activity-based

anorexia in mice. Clinical Nutrition. 2014;**33**(6):1046-1053

[87] Monteleone P et al. Intestinal permeability is decreased in anorexia nervosa. Molecular Psychiatry. 2004;**9**(1):76-80

[88] Pals KL et al. Effect of running intensity on intestinal permeability. Journal of Applied Physiology (Bethesda, MD: 1985). 1997;**82**(2):571-576

[89] Kishi T, Elmquist JK. Body weight is regulated by the brain: A link between feeding and emotion. Molecular Psychiatry. 2005;**10**(2):132-146

[90] Raevuori A et al. The increased risk for autoimmune diseases in patients with eating disorders. PLoS One. 2014;**9**(8):e104845

[91] Devkota S et al. Dietary-fat-induced taurocholic acid promotes pathobiont expansion and colitis in Il10−/− mice. Nature. 2012;**487**(7405):104-108

Section 3

Patients and Their Carers: Different Perspectives and Family Support

Chapter 7

Patients' and Carers' Perspectives of Psychopharmacological Interventions Targeting Anorexia Nervosa Symptoms

Amabel Dessain, Jessica Bentley, Janet Treasure, Ulrike Schmidt and Hubertus Himmerich

Abstract

In clinical practice, patients with anorexia nervosa (AN), their carers and clinicians often disagree about psychopharmacological treatment. We developed two corresponding questionnaires to survey the perspectives of patients with AN and their carers on psychopharmacological treatment. These questionnaires were distributed to 36 patients and 37 carers as a quality improvement project on a specialist unit for eating disorders at the South London and Maudsley NHS Foundation Trust. Although most patients did not believe that medication could help with AN, the majority thought that medication for AN should help with anxiety (61.1%), concentration (52.8%), sleep problems (52.8%) and anorexic thoughts (55.6%). Most of the carers shared the view that drug treatment for AN should help with anxiety (54%) and anorexic thoughts (64.8%). Most patients had concerns about potential weight gain, increased appetite, changes in body shape and metabolism during psychopharmacological treatment. By contrast, the majority of carers were not concerned about these specific side effects. Some of the concerns expressed by the patients seem to be AN-related. However, their desire for help with anxiety and anorexic thoughts, which is shared by their carers, should be taken seriously by clinicians when choosing a medication or planning psychopharmacological studies.

Keywords: anorexia nervosa, psychopharmacological treatment, treatment effects, side effects, opinion survey, patients, carers

1. Introduction

1.1 Anorexia nervosa

Anorexia nervosa (AN) is an eating disorder. According to the 5th edition of the Diagnostic and Statistical Manual of Mental Disorders (DSM-5) [1], its diagnostic criteria are significantly low body weight, intense fear of weight gain, and disturbed body perception. The prevalence of AN is up to 1% among women with a men-to-women ratio of 1–10 [2]. The peak incidence is at an age between 14 and 17 years [3]. The course is often chronic, and it can lead to persistent disability [4]. A recent longitudinal cohort study showed that only about 30% of patients with AN have recovered after 9 years [5]. AN has also been reported to be associated with a significantly increased mortality with a standardized mortality ratio (SMR) of 5.21 [6]. Thus, novel approaches such as psychopharmacological options should be considered to improve the treatment outcome and the care for people with AN.

1.2 Carers' help for patients with anorexia nervosa

Family members, partners and friends are usually highly motivated to care for patients with AN, but they are also often suffering. AN can make them feel guilty or anxious which is neither justified nor helpful. Family therapy for AN can tackle these feelings, can identify interpersonal difficulties maintaining the disorder, teach psychosocial and communication skills, and thus enable the carers to help the patients work towards recovery [7, 8]. The carers' help may also include supporting psychopharmacological treatment.

1.3 Psychopharmacological treatment for anorexia nervosa

The discovery of psychopharmacological treatment options in the 1950s led to a massive breakthrough in the treatment of schizophrenia and depression. Patients who previously had to live in asylums became enabled to lead a self-determined and autonomous life with their families, and resume taking up employment [9]. Patients with AN, however, did not benefit from this success, as the antipsychotics and antidepressants developed did not prove to be effective in AN.

Psychiatric researchers have unsuccessfully tried for decades to apply these medications to the treatment of AN, which is why there is no single medication approved for use in AN [10]. Part of the problem is the difficulty in conducting randomized controlled trials (RCTs) in AN. Most of these RCTs chose weight gain as their main outcome criterion. However, this is what patients with AN fear, and this fear is indeed a symptom of their disorder. Therefore, recruitment for psychopharmacological studies in AN has been a significant challenge [11]. Despite these obstacles, RCTs have been performed and published, although the recruitment rate of these RCTs has been so low that the results may not be generalizable.

The lack of effective psychopharmacological treatment has left patients with AN in a situation where clinical treatment outcomes are very modest. End-of-treatment remission rates of RCTs in adult patients with AN range between 13 and 43% [12]. This is a sobering figure highlighting the pernicious nature of AN and its mortality rate, which is—as already mentioned above—five to six times greater than in the general population [6, 13, 14].

The biological mechanisms leading to AN are not completely understood. Therefore, currently it is not possible to design a drug that would specifically target the biological cause of this psychiatric disorder [10]. However, clinicians could consider prescribing medication that targets certain symptoms which are important or frequent in patients with AN.

1.4 The patients' perspective

During the psychiatric history taking and examination, patients with AN often report that they use self-starvation to cope with stress, difficulties and overwhelming emotions. Thus, AN could be seen as a strategy for coping with underlying problems such as stress, anxiety or low mood [15]. Therefore, a medication that induces appetite and increases weight could be perceived by patients with AN as a way of re-exposing them to these underlying problems. Therefore, when drug treatment is considered, patients with AN are more interested in whether this medication might help with certain psychological symptoms including anxiety, mood, and problems with concentration and sleep [10, 16].

Weight gain can thus only be a first treatment step to reverse the acute effects of starvation. Relying on weight outcomes alone in drawing conclusions from RCTs could inflate the interpretation of positive results [14]. Instead, weight gain and psychological improvement should be considered as important treatment outcomes in their own right [14].

Psychopharmacological agents have potential side effects, including an increase in appetite, weight gain, binge eating, alterations in metabolism, cardiac problems, nausea, haematological changes, tiredness, mood changes and other psychological effects. It is important to share these potential side effects with the patients when obtaining their consent to treatment, as sharing this knowledge helps the process of shared decision-making about a psychopharmacological treatment and contributes to drug safety [17, 18].

1.5 The carers' perspective

As carers can support their loved ones towards recovery [19], it makes sense to involve them in medical and specifically psychopharmacological decisions. They can support patients when they take their medication, and they can observe and report beneficial and adverse effects. Thus, we surveyed the carers' views and expectations towards psychopharmacological treatment for AN. In this chapter, the term 'carer' is used quite broadly. It can be anyone caring for a person with an eating disorder, such as a parent, a sibling, a partner or a friend.

1.6 Aim of this study

This study was performed to survey the patients' and carers' perspectives of psychopharmacological interventions targeting symptoms of AN. Therefore, a questionnaire was developed to gather the patients' views and another questionnaire, with questions of similar content, was developed to gather the carers' views. In this book chapter, we present both these questionnaires on the patients' and the carers' views on psychopharmacological treatment for AN, and we report on the statistical results of the survey.

2. Methods

2.1 Development of the questionnaires

In order to perform a quality improvement (QI) project in the Eating Disorders Service of the South London and Maudsley NHS Foundation Trust (SLaM), we developed a questionnaire for such a project. The QI project team consisted of patients and psychiatrists from the eating disorders inpatient ward, the 'step-up' service (a day-hospital service) and the outpatient unit of SLaM. The questionnaire has three main sections. The first section provides basic information on the patient or the carer and their experience with medication prescribed to them or their loved one respectively. The second section asks about what therapeutic effects a psychopharmacological medication should have to help with symptoms of AN. The third section is about concerns of potential side effects.

Initially, the questionnaires were distributed to a group of 17 patients with AN and 16 carers between June 2016 and January 2017. The answers given were evaluated and the main results have been published in a scientific letter [16]. The feedback received from SLaM patients, carers and colleagues suggested minor alterations to the wording of a few questions and the addition of three further questions. Therefore, we made these changes accordingly and distributed the questionnaires to a second cohort of 19 patients and 21 carers between March and September 2018. Thus, taking both cohorts together, we obtained completed questionnaires from 36 patients and 37 carers.

The patient and the carer questionnaires used in the second cohort are depicted in the appendix of this article.

2.2 Study sample

The total sample of people who completed the questionnaires included 36 patients and 37 carers.

Patients were all females between 18 and 44 years of age; mean age: 27.64 years ± 6.85 standard deviation (SD); seven were treated as outpatients, five as day-patients and 24 as inpatients in our specialist unit at the time of the survey. The duration of treatment ranged between 1 week and 15 years; mean duration of treatment: 50.12 weeks ± 136.62 SD. The duration of their AN was between 1 year and 24 years; mean 9.03 years ± 6.67 SD. Twenty-four of these patients were currently receiving psychopharmacological treatment.

The carers were 21 males and 16 females between 21 and 71 years; mean age: 51.40 years ± 11.11 SD. Their close others with AN were two male and 35 female patients between 18 and 44 years old, mean age: 24.62 years ± 6.71 SD. Of these close others with AN, 12 were treated as outpatients, three as day-patients and 22 as inpatients in our unit at the time of the survey. The duration of treatment of these patients ranged from 'not yet started' to 52 weeks; mean duration of treatment: 11.60 weeks ± 12.20 SD. The duration of their AN was between 1 and 20 years; mean 7.01 years ± 6.64 SD. A total of 27 of these patients were currently on medication for mental health problems.

2.3 Data evaluation and statistics

The questionnaires were statistically evaluated using IBM SPSS statistics version 24. We used descriptive statistics to evaluate the questionnaires.

For consistency, the additional questions in the new version of both the patients' and the carers' questionnaires were excluded from statistical evaluation. Thus, the questions on appetite increase and improved gastrointestinal symptoms as potentially desired effects of medication for AN were not included, nor was the question about concerns of changes in the way of thinking as a potential side effect. The evaluation of free text answers was not part of the current publication.

3. Results

3.1 Opinions about therapeutic effects of a medication for anorexia nervosa

Regarding the overall opinion on drug treatment for AN, most patients disagreed in our survey with the view that medication could help with AN, whereas the majority of carers were undecided in this regard. Approximately one third of patients were also neutral about this. In terms of the question on whether patients with AN should consider medication for treatment, a proportion of almost 40% of patients and carers expressed no particular point of view. However, more than half of the carers believed that patients with AN should consider drug treatment. Most of the patients agreed or strongly agreed with the statement that they did not want medication for treatment with AN, whereas the carers had more diverse opinions in this respect with ~40% of neutral opinion and 65% of carers believing that medication should be taken if recommended. However, patients were more cautious about this statement, with 42% expressing a neutral view on this.

The results revealed that ~50% of patients agreed or strongly agreed with each of the following target symptoms of psychopharmacological treatment: anxiety (61.1%; sum of 'agreed' plus 'strongly agreed'), concentration (52.8%), sleep problems (52.8%) and anorexic thoughts (55.6%). Most of the carers shared the view that drug treatment should help with anxiety (54%) and anorexic thoughts (64.8%).

In both patients and carers, ~75% stated that more research on drug treatment for AN is needed. As much as 40% of patients expressed their willingness to take part in such research, and ~25% of patients were undecided about whether they should take part or not.

Detailed information on the frequencies and percentages of answers concerning the therapeutic effects of a medication for the treatment of AN can be found in **Table 1**.

3.2 Concerns about side effects of medication for anorexia nervosa

More than 90% of patients agreed or strongly agreed that they had concerns about potential weight gain during psychopharmacological treatment, and about the same number of patients also expressed concerns about appetite increase during drug treatment. Furthermore, the majority of patients were afraid of binge eating, changes in body shape and changes in metabolism.

Most of the patients were also concerned about potential side effects not related to appetite or weight regulation. These included changes in mood, tiredness or sleepiness, problems with the heart or the heart rhythm, nausea, decreased concentration, changes in laboratory parameters and sleep problems.

By contrast, a majority of carers were not concerned about weight gain, appetite increase, and changes in body shape nor metabolism. However, most of the carers feared binge eating as a side effect and adverse effects related to mood, tiredness, heart problems, nausea, concentration, laboratory parameters and sleep.

Detailed information on frequencies and percentages of answers concerning the potential side effects of a medication for the treatment of AN can be found in **Table 2**.

4. Discussion

4.1 Summary of findings

Taken together, we have developed questionnaires for patients with AN and for carers to express their opinion on psychopharmacological treatment for AN. Most patients did not think that medication could help with AN. However, the majority of patients thought that medication for AN should help with anxiety, concentration, sleep problems and anorexic thoughts. In this respect, most of the carers shared the view that drug treatment for AN should help with anxiety and anorexic thoughts. Almost all patients who participated in the survey had concerns about potential weight gain and increased appetite during psychopharmacological treatment, and most of them also feared changes in body shape and metabolism. The majority of

	Patients (N = 36)		Carers (N = 37)	
	Frequency	Percent (%)	Frequency	Percent (%)
Medication could help with anorexia nervosa				
Strongly disagree	1	2.8	0	0
Disagree	18	50.0	1	2.7
Neutral	11	30.6	21	56.8
Agree	6	16.7	12	32.4
Strongly agree	0	0	2	5.4
Patients with anorexia nervosa should consider medication for treatment				
Strongly disagree	3	8.3	0	0
Disagree	5	13.9	1	2.7
Neutral	14	38.9	14	37.8
Agree	12	33.3	20	54.1
Strongly agree	2	5.6	1	2.7
I do not want medication for anorexia nervosa				
Strongly disagree	2	5.6	7	18.9
Disagree	8	22.2	8	21.6
Neutral	7	19.4	14	37.8
Agree	14	38.9	6	16.2
Strongly agree	5	13.9	1	2.7
Medication should be taken if recommended				
Strongly disagree	1	2.8	0	0
Disagree	3	8.3	0	0
Neutral	15	41.7	10	27.0
Agree	16	44.4	24	64.9
Strongly agree	1	2.8	1	2.7
Medication should help with anxiety				
Strongly disagree	2	5.6	0	0
Disagree	4	11.1	3	8.1
Neutral	8	22.2	11	29.7
Agree	16	44.4	17	45.9
Strongly agree	6	16.7	3	8.1
Medication should help with low mood				
Strongly disagree	3	8.3	0	0
Disagree	7	19.4	3	8.1
Neutral	9	25.0	15	40.5
Agree	8	22.2	14	37.8
Strongly agree	9	25.0	3	8.1

	Patients (N = 36)		Carers (N = 37)	
	Frequency	**Percent (%)**	**Frequency**	**Percent (%)**
Medication should help to improve concentration				
Strongly disagree	1	2.8	1	2.7
Disagree	9	25.0	6	16.2
Neutral	7	19.4	17	45.9
Agree	14	38.9	9	24.3
Strongly agree	5	13.9	2	5.4
Medication should help with sleep				
Strongly disagree	1	2.8	1	2.7
Disagree	4	11.1	3	8.1
Neutral	12	33.3	17	45.9
Agree	11	30.6	10	27.0
Strongly agree	8	22.2	3	8.1
Medication should weaken anorexic thoughts				
Strongly disagree	1	2.8	0	0
Disagree	3	8.3	2	5.4
Neutral	12	33.3	9	24.3
Agree	15	41.7	18	48.6
Strongly agree	5	13.9	6	16.2
More research on drug treatment for anorexia nervosa is needed				
Strongly disagree	0	0	1	2.7
Disagree	1	2.8	0	0
Neutral	7	19.4	5	13.5
Agree	14	38.9	13	35.1
Strongly agree	13	36.1	15	40.5
Willingness to take part in research for drug treatment for anorexia nervosa				
Strongly disagree	5	13.9	2	5.4
Disagree	7	19.4	6	16.2
Neutral	10	27.8	18	48.6
Agree	8	22.2	7	18.9
Strongly agree	6	16.7	2	5.4

For the exact wording of the questions, see questionnaire 1 and 2 in the appendix of this chapter.

Table 1.
Frequencies and percentages of answers regarding the overall opinion on drug treatment for AN, important target symptoms, relevance of psychopharmacological research and willingness to take part.

carers, in contrast, was not concerned about weight gain, appetite increase, changes in body shape and metabolism. All the addressed side effects were of concern to patients. For the carers, for most of the questions on side effects, between 20 and 40% of had no particular opinion and thus gave a neutral answer.

	Patients (N = 36)		Carers (N = 37)	
	Frequency	**Percent (%)**	**Frequency**	**Percent (%)**
Concerns about weight gain during drug treatment				
Strongly disagree	0	0	3	8.1
Disagree	1	2.8	10	27.0
Neutral	2	5.6	11	29.7
Agree	9	25.0	6	16.2
Strongly agree	24	66.7	5	13.5
Concerns about appetite increase during drug treatment				
Strongly disagree	0	0	2	5.4
Disagree	2	5.6	11	29.7
Neutral	1	2.8	13	35.1
Agree	13	36.1	3	8.1
Strongly agree	20	55.6	4	10.8
Concerns about binge eating during drug treatment				
Strongly disagree	1	2.8	1	2.7
Disagree	2	5.6	1	2.7
Neutral	3	8.3	7	18.9
Agree	8	22.2	13	35.1
Strongly agree	22	61.1	10	27.0
Concerns about changes in body shape during drug treatment				
Strongly disagree	1	2.8	2	5.4
Disagree	0	0	5	13.5
Neutral	2	5.6	17	45.9
Agree	14	38.9	4	10.8
Strongly agree	19	52.8	4	10.8
Concerns about changes in metabolism during drug treatment				
Strongly disagree	0	0	1	2.7
Disagree	1	2.8	4	10.8
Neutral	2	5.6	14	37.8
Agree	11	30.6	9	24.3
Strongly agree	22	61.1	5	13.5
Concerns about mood changes during drug treatment				
Strongly disagree	1	2.8	0	0
Disagree	1	2.8	2	5.4
Neutral	4	11.1	6	16.2
Agree	18	50.0	18	48.6
Strongly agree	12	33.3	8	21.6

	Patients (N = 36)		Carers (N = 37)	
	Frequency	**Percent (%)**	**Frequency**	**Percent (%)**
Concerns about tiredness or sleepiness during drug treatment				
Strongly disagree	0	0	1	2.7
Disagree	3	8.3	2	5.4
Neutral	8	22.2	8	21.6
Agree	14	38.9	16	43.2
Strongly agree	11	30.6	7	18.9
Concerns about problems with the heart or the heart rhythm				
Strongly disagree	1	2.8	0	0
Disagree	1	2.8	0	0
Neutral	10	27.8	3	8.1
Agree	14	38.9	8	21.6
Strongly agree	10	27.8	23	62.2
Concerns about nausea during drug treatment				
Strongly disagree	0	0	0	0
Disagree	3	8.3	1	2.7
Neutral	12	33.3	5	13.5
Agree	14	38.9	18	48.6
Strongly agree	7	19.4	10	27.0
Concerns about decreased concentration during drug treatment				
Strongly disagree	0	0	0	0
Disagree	0	0	0	0
Neutral	8	22.2	10	27.0
Agree	16	44.4	15	40.5
Strongly agree	12	33.3	10	27.0
Concerns about changes in laboratory parameters during drug treatment				
Strongly disagree	1	2.8	1	2.7
Disagree	4	11.1	1	2.7
Neutral	12	33.3	6	16.2
Agree	12	33.3	15	40.5
Strongly agree	7	19.4	11	29.7
Concerns about sleep problems during drug treatment				
Strongly disagree	0	0	1	2.7
Disagree	1	2.8	0	0
Neutral	3	8.3	4	10.8
Agree	19	52.8	20	54.1
Strongly agree	12	33.3	10	27.0

For the exact wording of the questions, see questionnaire 1 and 2 in the appendix of this chapter.

Table 2.
Frequencies and percentages of answers regarding the overall opinion on side effects of drug treatment for AN.

4.2 Patients perspective on medication—not suitable to treat anorexia nervosa but of concern because of weight gain as a side effect

The most obvious discrepancy within the patients' answers is that they did not believe medication could help with AN, and were at the same time concerned about appetite increase and weight gain as potential side effects of medication. This finding is of great relevance, as the primary outcome criterion in the majority of clinical studies in AN is an increase in body weight [10, 11, 20]. However, patients may not perceive weight gain as the core problem of AN, because—as stated earlier—self-starvation is their own way to attenuate negative affective states and aversive emotions [12]. Therefore, drug treatment to gain weight alone cannot be perceived as a good treatment option from the patients' perspective.

It is of course necessary for patients with AN to gain weight due to the medical risk associated with extremely low body weight. However, this weight gain should be supported by addressing the underlying difficulties of anxiety and anorexic thoughts.

4.3 Anxiety and anorexic thoughts as outcome parameters for future treatment studies

Our survey showed that anxiety is an important symptom that patients with AN and their carers want to be addressed during psychopharmacological therapy. This is not unexpected, as AN has been found to be closely associated with anxiety disorders [21].

Therefore, questionnaires for anxiety and depression should be used to measure the outcome of RCTs in AN. However, there are many different questionnaires available, which all have their advantages and disadvantages. Thus, the suggestions below may seem arbitrary, however, we would like to provide the reader with some specific suggestions as to how anxiety, depression and anorexic psychopathology can be measured.

The Brief Psychiatric Rating Scale (BPRS) assesses 24 different psychiatric symptoms, among them anxiety, depression, unusual thought content and emotional withdrawal [22]. The Depression Anxiety Stress Scales (DASS) is an instrument designed to measure the three related negative emotional states of depression, anxiety and stress [23]. There is a 21-item as well as a 42-item available. Both these questionnaires could be applied in clinical practice to measure the level of anxiety in a patient with AN or used in future RCTs to test psychopharmacological therapies with regard to their effectiveness in reducing anxiety. In children, the Revised Children's Anxiety and Depression Scale (RCADS), a 47-item questionnaire that measures the frequency of various symptoms of anxiety and low mood, may be used [24]. However, our study sample did not include children and adolescents.

To measure anorexic thoughts, the Yale-Brown-Cornell Eating Disorders Scale (YBC-EDS) [25], the Eating Disorder Examination-Questionnaire (EDE-Q) [26] and the Revised Beliefs about Voices Questionnaire (BAVQ-R) [27], could be used. The YBC-EDS measures core preoccupations and rituals related to eating disorders, the EDE-Q assesses key behavioural features and associated psychopathology of eating disorders and the BAVQ-R is a self-reported measure of patients' beliefs, emotions and behaviour about auditory hallucinations.

4.4 Information on pharmacological treatments for patients and carers

The fact that a large proportion of patients and carers were neutral about certain statements regarding psychopharmacological treatment for AN is not surprising, as currently no medication is approved for the treatment of AN [10]. Therefore, clinicians could abstain from using psychopharmacological treatment at all and also from informing patients about this opportunity. However, there is positive evidence from clinical studies for a few drugs, and clinicians may share the results of these studies with their patients and carers.

For example, olanzapine was found to be superior to placebo in four published RCTs [28–31] in AN regarding weight gain. It has also been shown to have a beneficial influence on anxiety [32, 33] and sleep [34] in patients with psychosis. Helping with anxiety and sleep were important features of a psychopharmacological drug for patients with AN in our survey. Thus, the high number of people giving a neutral answer in our survey may point to the need for more information to be shared with patients and their carers about the psychopharmacological options.

4.5 Side effects

Most patients had concerns about potential weight gain, increased appetite, and changes in body shape and metabolism. This is understandable, because these are AN-related fears.

However, the last three decades have seen substantial scientific efforts to examine the metabolic side effects of psychopharmacological agents, specifically antipsychotic agents. Weight gain, high blood glucose levels, impaired insulin sensitivity and changes in lipid metabolism have been found to be unfavourable [35]. However, these results were first and foremost obtained in patients with schizophrenia. In patients with AN, however, we have a diametrically opposite metabolic 'starting situation' compared to patients with schizophrenia, as AN patients are significantly underweight, are at risk of severe hypoglycaemia and hypertriglyceridemia, and have been found to have an increased insulin sensitivity [36, 37]. Therefore, the side effects of certain antipsychotics, including olanzapine which increase blood glucose levels, lower insulin sensitivity, elevate triglyceride levels and lead to weight gain [35], do appear to be less problematic in patients with AN.

The evidence from RCTs, however, is insufficient in AN to make firm recommendations; and there are no medications approved for the treatment of AN. Therefore, the above-mentioned conclusions should be drawn with caution, even though they may appear obvious.

4.6 Limitations

Our survey has several limitations. First of all, the applied questionnaires were developed during this QI project and are not established measures for examining patients' and carers' opinions on psychopharmacological treatment. At approximately halfway through the study, we decided to make some minor amendments to the questionnaires, which led to constraints in the statistical evaluation of the survey. Secondly, the sample size of 36 patients and 37 carers is relatively low. However, we hope that by sharing the questionnaires in this book chapter, other scientists will use them for their research which will lead to a broader database. Thirdly, a major shortcoming of this survey is the inclusion of adult patients with AN only, whereas AN is a disorder that starts in childhood and adolescence.

5. Conclusion

We developed two corresponding questionnaires to survey the perspectives of people with AN and their carers on psychopharmacological treatment for AN.

Although most patients did not believe that medication could help with AN, the majority thought that medication for AN should help with anxiety, concentration, sleep problems and anorexic thoughts. Most of the carers shared the view that drug treatment for AN should help with anxiety and anorexic thoughts. Therefore, these symptoms should be given attention when prescribing psychopharmacological agents for people with AN or when planning RCTs for AN.

Most patients had concerns about potential weight gain, increased appetite, changes in body shape and metabolism. However, psychopharmacological drugs may actually help with metabolic peculiarities in patients with AN, including hypoglycaemia.

No psychopharmacological treatment is currently approved for AN, and scientific data on effects and side effects in individuals with AN is scarce. Therefore, although far-reaching conclusions should not be drawn, the available data and information should be shared with patients and their carers to reach the best possible decision on whether drugs should be used for the treatment of AN.

Acknowledgements

The authors would like to thank all patients, carers and colleagues at the South London and Maudsley NHS Foundation Trust and King's College London, who were involved in the fruitful and helpful discussions concerning the development of the questionnaires.

Conflict of interest

The authors declare that there is no conflict of interest.

Appendix. Questionnaires

A.1 Questionnaire 1: patient views on medication targeting anorexia nervosa symptoms

This questionnaire has been created to help develop research around the use of psychopharmacological medication in anorexia nervosa. Your input will help refine future research projects. Please answer the questions according to what you think. Insert own text if required. Thank you for your participation.

Personal information

1.	My age	Years
2.	My gender	Female/male/other

3. My current treatment: I am currently treated in the following service (FREED, Outpatient, Day-care, SEED, Step-up, Inpatient):

4. Duration of my current treatment in the above-mentioned service:

Duration of illness

5. For how many years have you had anorexia nervosa?

	Years

Previous drug treatment for anorexia nervosa

	Yes	No
6. I have been treated with a psychiatric medication (medication for your mental health).		
7. I have been treated with antipsychotic medication (such as olanzapine, quetiapine).		
8. I have been treated with antidepressant medication (such as sertraline, fluoxetine).		

9. Are you currently taking/have you previously taken prescribed medication relating to anorexia nervosa? Please specify which.

10. Have you experienced side effects from this medication? Please specify.

11. Do you feel the medication helped?

Opinion about therapeutic effects of a medication for anorexia nervosa

	Strongly disagree	Disagree	Neutral	Agree	Strongly agree
12. I think a drug could help treat my anorexia nervosa.					
13. I would consider taking medication for treatment of anorexia nervosa.					
14. I don't want to take any medication.					
15. I would take medication if it is recommended by my therapist or medical doctor.					
16. I would like medication to help me with my anxiety.					
17. I would like medication to help me with my mood.					
18. I would like medication to help improve my concentration.					
19. I would like medication to help increase my appetite.					
20. I would like a medication to help improve my sleep.					
21. I would like a medication to help me with gastrointestinal symptoms such as constipation.					
22. I would like medication to help weaken the anorexic voice or anorexic thoughts.					

	Strongly disagree	Disagree	Neutral	Agree	Strongly agree
23. There should be more research on drug treatments in anorexia nervosa.					
24. I would take part in a trial to assist in research into drug treatment for anorexia nervosa.					

25. In your own words, what else would you like medication to help with in overcoming anorexia nervosa?

Views on side effects of a medication for anorexia nervosa

Which of the following potential side effects would you be concerned about in taking a new medication?

	Strongly disagree	Disagree	Neutral	Agree	Strongly agree
26. Weight gain					
27. Appetite increase					
28. Binge eating					
29. Changes in my body shape					
30. My metabolism could change, making it harder to burn calories					
31. Mood changes					
32. Tiredness or sleepiness					
33. Problems with my heart or heart rhythm.					
34. Nausea					
35. Decreased concentration					
36. Changes in my bloods					
37. Sleep problems					
38. Changes in the way you think					

39. In your own words: What side effect do you fear most?

40. Further comments and suggestions for research around medication targeting anorexia nervosa symptoms.

Thank you for taking part in this survey and answering the questions.

A.2 Questionnaire 2: carer views on medication targeting anorexia nervosa symptoms

This questionnaire has been created to help develop research around the use of psychopharmacological medication in anorexia nervosa. Your input will help refine future research projects. Please answer the questions according to what you think. Insert own text if required. Thank you for your participation.

Personal information

1.	My own age	Years
2.	My own gender	Female/male/other
3.	Age of my loved one with anorexia nervosa	Years
4.	Gender of my loved one with anorexia nervosa	Female/male/other

5. Current treatment: My loved one is currently receiving eating disorder treatment in the following service (FREED, Outpatient, Day-care, SEED, Step-up, Inpatient):

6. Duration of my loved one's current treatment in the above-mentioned service:

Duration of illness

7. For how many years has your loved one had anorexia nervosa?

Years

Previous drug treatment for anorexia nervosa

		Yes	No
8.	My loved one has been treated with medication for their mental health problem.		
9.	My loved one has been treated with antipsychotic medication (such as olanzapine, quetiapine).		
10.	My loved one has been treated with antidepressant medication (such as sertraline, fluoxetine).		

11. Is your loved one currently taking/has your loved one previously taken prescribed medication relating to anorexia nervosa or other mental health problems? Please specify which.

12. Has your loved one experienced side effects from this medication? Please specify.

13. Do you feel the medication helped them?

Opinion about therapeutic effects of a medication for anorexia nervosa

		Strongly disagree	Disagree	Neutral	Agree	Strongly agree
14.	I think medication could help my loved one with anorexia nervosa.					
15.	Patients with anorexia nervosa should consider taking medication for treatment of anorexia nervosa.					
16.	I don't want my loved one to take medication.					

	Strongly disagree	Disagree	Neutral	Agree	Strongly agree
17. My loved one should take medication if it is recommended by a therapist or medical doctor.					
18. I would want any medication to help my loved one with their anxiety.					
19. I would want any medication to help my loved one with their low mood.					
20. I would want any medication to help my loved one improve their concentration.					
21. I would want any medication to help my loved one increase their appetite.					
22. I would want any medication to help my loved one to sleep better.					
23. I would want any medication to help my loved one with gastrointestinal symptoms such as constipation.					
24. I would want any medication to help weaken the anorexic voice or anorexic thoughts my loved one was experiencing.					
25. There should be more research on drug treatments in anorexia nervosa.					
26. I would encourage my loved one to take part in a clinical trial on drug treatment for anorexia nervosa.					

27. In your own words, what else would you like medication to help your loved one with in overcoming anorexia nervosa?

Views on side effects of a medication for anorexia nervosa

Which of the following potential side effects would you be concerned about, if your loved one takes medication?

	Strongly disagree	Disagree	Neutral	Agree	Strongly agree
28. Weight gain					
29. Appetite increase					
30. Binge eating					
31. Changes in body shape					
32. The metabolism could change, making it harder to burn calories					
33. Mood changes					
34. Tiredness or sleepiness					
35. Problems with the heart or heart rhythm.					
36. Nausea					
37. Decreased concentration					
38. Changes in bloods					

	Strongly disagree	Disagree	Neutral	Agree	Strongly agree
39. Sleep problems					
40. Changes in the way they think					

41. In your own words: What side effect do you fear most for your loved one?

42. Further comments and suggestions for research around medication targeting anorexia nervosa symptoms.

Thank you for taking part in this survey and answering the questions.

Author details

Amabel Dessain[1*], Jessica Bentley[2], Janet Treasure[1,2], Ulrike Schmidt[1,2] and Hubertus Himmerich[1,2]

1 South London and Maudsley NHS Foundation Trust, London, UK

2 Department of Psychological Medicine, King's College London, London, UK

*Address all correspondence to: amabel.dessain@slam.nhs.uk

References

[1] American Psychiatric Association. Diagnostic and Statistical Manual of Mental Disorders. 5th ed. Arlington, VA: APA Publishing; 2013

[2] Keski-Rahkonen A, Mustelin L. Epidemiology of eating disorders in Europe: Prevalence, incidence, comorbidity, course, consequences, and risk factors. Current Opinion in Psychiatry. 2016;**29**:340-345. DOI: 10.1097/YCO.0000000000000278

[3] Javaras KN, Runfola CD, Thornton LM, et al. Sex- and age-specific incidence of healthcare-register-recorded eating disorders in the complete Swedish 1979-2001 birth cohort. The International Journal of Eating Disorders. 2015;**48**:1070-1081. DOI: 10.1002/eat.22467

[4] Schmidt U, Adan R, Böhm I, Campbell IC, Dingemans A, Ehrlich S, et al. Eating disorders: The big issue. Lancet Psychiatry. 2016;**3**:313-315. DOI: 10.1016/S2215-0366(16)00081-X

[5] Eddy KT, Tabri N, Thomas JJ, Murray HB, Keshaviah A, Hastings E, et al. Recovery from anorexia nervosa and bulimia nervosa at 22-year follow-up. Journal of Clinical Psychiatry. 2017; **78**:184-189. DOI: 10.4088/JCP.15m10393

[6] Himmerich H, Hotopf M, Shetty H, Schmidt U, Treasure J, Hayes RD, et al. Psychiatric comorbidity as a risk factor for mortality in people with anorexia nervosa. European Archives of Psychiatry and Clinical Neuroscience. 2019;**269**:351-359. DOI: 10.1007/s00406-018-0937-8

[7] Rienecke RD. Family-based treatment of eating disorders in adolescents: Current insights. Adolescent Health, Medicine and Therapeutics. 2017;**8**:69-79. DOI: 10.2147/AHMT.S115775

[8] Chen EY, Weissman JA, Zeffiro TA, Yiu A, Eneva KT, Arlt JM, et al. Family-based therapy for young adults with anorexia nervosa restores weight. The International Journal of Eating Disorders. 2016;**49**:701-707. DOI: 10.1002/eat.22513

[9] Thuillier J. Ten years which changed psychiatry. In: Healy D, editor. The Psychopharmacologists. London: Arnold; 2000. pp. 543-559

[10] Himmerich H, Treasure J. Psychopharmacological advances in eating disorders. Expert Review in Clinical Pharmacology. 2018;**11**:95-108. DOI: 10.1080/17512433.2018.1383895

[11] Miniati M, Mauri M, Ciberti A, Mariani MG, Marazziti D, Dell'Osso L. Psychopharmacological options for adult patients with anorexia nervosa. CNS Spectrums. 2016;**21**:134-142. DOI: 10.1017/S1092852914000790

[12] Brockmeyer T, Friederich HC, Schmidt U. Advances in the treatment of anorexia nervosa: A review of established and emerging interventions. Psychological Medicine. 2018;**48**: 1228-1256. DOI: 10.1017/S0033291717002604

[13] Arcelus J, Mitchell AJ, Wales J, Nielsen S. Mortality rates in patients with anorexia nervosa and other eating disorders. A meta-analysis of 36 studies. Archives of General Psychiatry. 2011;**68**: 724-731. DOI: 10.1001/archgenpsychiatry.2011.74

[14] Murray SB, Loeb KL, Le Grange D. Treatment outcome reporting in anorexia nervosa: Time for a paradigm shift? Journal of Eating Disorders. 2018; **6**:10. DOI: 10.1186/s40337-018-0195-1

[15] Brockmeyer T, Holtforth MG, Bents H, Kämmerer A, Herzog W, Friederich

HC. Starvation and emotion regulation in anorexia nervosa. Comprehensive Psychiatry. 2012;**53**:496-501. DOI: 10.1016/j.comppsych.2011.09.003

[16] Himmerich H, Joaquim M, Bentley J, Kan C, Dornik J, Treasure J, et al. Psychopharmacological options for adult patients with anorexia nervosa: The patients' and carers' perspectives. CNS Spectrums. 2018;**23**:251-252. DOI: 10.1017/S1092852917000529

[17] Stübner S, Grohmann R, Schmauß M. Drug safety in clinical practice—Part 1: Psychopharmacological treatment. Fortschritte der Neurologie-Psychiatrie. 2012;**80**:468-480. DOI: 10.1055/s-0032-1313085

[18] Stübner S, Grohmann R, Schmauß M. Drug safety in clinical practice—Part 2: Psychopharmacological treatment. Fortschritte der Neurologie-Psychiatrie. 2013;**81**:715-727. DOI: 10.1055/s-0033-1355883

[19] Treasure J, Nazar BP. Interventions for the carers of patients with eating disorders. Current Psychiatry Reports. 2016;**18**:16. DOI: 10.1007/s11920-015-0652-3

[20] Dold M, Aigner M, Klabunde M, Treasure J, Kasper S. Second-generation antipsychotic drugs in anorexia nervosa: A meta-analysis of randomized controlled trials. Psychotherapy and Psychosomatics. 2015;**84**:110-116. DOI: 10.1159/000369978

[21] Godart NT, Flament MF, Perdereau F, Jeammet P. Comorbidity between eating disorders and anxiety disorders: A review. The International Journal of Eating Disorders. 2002;**32**:253-270. DOI: 10.1002/eat.10096

[22] Overall JE, Gorham DR. The brief psychiatric rating scale. Psychological Reports. 1962;**10**:799-812

[23] Brown TA, Chorpita BF, Korotitsch W, Barlow DH. Psychometric properties of the depression anxiety stress scales (DASS) in clinical samples. Behaviour Research and Therapy. 1997;**35**:79-89

[24] Chorpita BF, Moffitt CE, Gray J. Psychometric properties of the revised child anxiety and depression scale in a clinical sample. Behaviour Research and Therapy. 2005;**43**:309-322. DOI: 10.1016/j.brat.2004.02.004

[25] Mazure CM, Halmi KA, Sunday SR, Romano SJ, Einhorn AM. The Yale-Brown-Cornell eating disorder scale: Development, use, reliability and validity. Journal of Psychiatric Research. 1994;**28**:425-445. DOI: 10.1016/0022-3956(94)90002-7

[26] Luce KH, Crowther JH. The reliability of the eating disorder examination-self-report questionnaire version (EDE-Q). The International Journal of Eating Disorders. 1999;**25**: 349-351. DOI: 10.1002/(SICI)1098-108X(199904)25:3<349::AID-EAT15>3.0.CO;2-M

[27] Chandwick P, Lees S, Birchwood M. The revised beliefs about voices questionnaire (BAVQ-R). The British Journal of Psychiatry. 2000;**177**:229-232. DOI: 10.1192/bjp.177.3.229

[28] Kafantaris V, Leigh E, Hertz S, Berest A, Schebendach J, Sterling WM, et al. A placebo-controlled pilot study of adjunctive olanzapine for adolescents with anorexia nervosa. Journal of Child and Adolescent Psychopharmacology. 2011;**21**:207-212. DOI: 10.1089/cap.2010.0139

[29] Brambilla F, Garcia CS, Fassino S, Daga GA, Favaro A, Santonastaso P, et al. Olanzapine therapy in anorexia nervosa: Psychobiological effects. International Clinical Psychopharmacology. 2007;**22**:197-204. DOI: 10.1097/YIC.0b013e328080ca31

[30] Bissada H, Tasca GA, Barber AM, Bradwejn J. Olanzapine in the treatment of low body weight and obsessive thinking in women with anorexia nervosa: A randomized, double-blind, placebo-controlled trial. American Journal of Psychiatry. 2008;**165**: 1281-1288. DOI: 10.1176/appi.ajp.2008.07121900

[31] Attia E, Kaplan AS, Walsh BT, Gershkovich M, Yilmaz Z, Musante D, et al. Olanzapine versus placebo for out-patients with anorexia nervosa. Psychological Medicine. 2011;**41**: 2177-2182. DOI: 10.1017/S0033291711000390

[32] Tollefson GD, Sanger TM. Anxious-depressive symptoms in schizophrenia: A new treatment target for pharmacotherapy? Schizophrenia Research. 1999;**1**(35 Suppl):13-21. DOI: 10.1016/S0920-9964(98)00164-9

[33] Temmingh H, Stein DJ. Anxiety in patients with schizophrenia: Epidemiology and management. CNS Drugs. 2015;**29**:819-832. DOI: 10.1007/s40263-015-0282-7

[34] Kluge M, Schacht A, Himmerich H, Rummel-Kluge C, Wehmeier PM, Dalal M, et al. Olanzapine and clozapine differently affect sleep in patients with schizophrenia: Results from a double-blind, polysomnographic study and review of the literature. Schizophrenia Research. 2014;**152**:255-260. DOI: 10.1016/j.schres.2013.11.009

[35] Himmerich H, Minkwitz J, Kirkby KC. Weight gain and metabolic changes during treatment with antipsychotics and antidepressants. Endocrine, Metabolic & Immune Disorders Drug Targets. 2015;**15**:252-260. DOI: 10.2174/1871530315666150623092031

[36] Ilyas A, Hübel C, Stahl D, Stadler M, Ismail K, Breen G, et al. The metabolic underpinning of eating disorders: A systematic review and meta-analysis of insulin sensitivity. Molecular and Cellular Endocrinology. 2018. DOI: 10.1016/j.mce.2018.10.005

[37] Winston AP. The clinical biochemistry of anorexia nervosa. Annals of Clinical Biochemistry. 2012; **49**(Pt 2):132-143. DOI: 10.1258/acb.2011.011185

Chapter 8

Storytelling as a Therapeutic Tool for Family Support in Bulimia Nervosa

José Vicente Martínez Quiñones, Mar Martínez Gamarra and Ignacio Jáuregui Lobera

Abstract

Telling stories (storytelling) is, above and beyond, a form of communication. It is a natural, universal, and well-known way of interaction among human beings. Storytelling, orally as well as in writing, is the sharing of personal narratives, a sort of story-sharing. With regard to chronic disease self-management, storytelling has been reported to be an exciting approach to patients and families. In this regard, families are considered very important in the management and treatment of eating disorders. Living with an eating disorder is an experience which deserves to be expressed in order to improve emotional support always necessary for patients' families. Bearing in mind that eating disorders can be chronic illnesses that lead to challenging and troublesome experiences for patients and their families, this chapter aims to think over the everyday interactions that typify family life in the context of eating disorders and specifically in the case of bulimia nervosa. We propose this text as a reflection based on different experiences when working with bulimic patients.

Keywords: storytelling, eating disorders, bulimia nervosa, family support, narratives

1. Introduction: what is storytelling?

Storytelling (ST) is a well-known tradition in human culture since people tend to tell stories for many reasons such as entertaining, transfer of knowledge between generations, maintenance of cultural heritage, warning others of dangers, etc. Telling stories with serious (non-entertainment) objectives has emerged as a new way for potential applications in different contexts (e.g., medicine or psychology) [1].

Above and beyond ST is a communication tool among human beings with a core aspect which is the emotions. "Serious" ST is an earnest narrative, a way to tell stories outside the context of entertainment. ST has different components such as narrative, perspective, interactivity, and medium. *Narrative* is the actual content of the story, which includes times-contexts, causes-effects, sequence, etc. *Perspective* refers to the fact that in each story the author conveys a subjective point of view of a certain aspect of the story. Perspective includes facets such as cognition, emotions, encoding-decoding, meaning, memory, etc. *Interactivity* is essential in ST, including story features such as engagement, modification/decision of narrative flow, etc. Finally, *medium* includes mediation, channels, forms, etc. When ST is defined as a narrative, two components must be considered: the narrative content (story) and the narrative form (discourse). Stories and discourses build a fundamental way for humans to make sense of the world (**Table 1**) [2].

Serious ST refers to a non-entertainment context, where stories are part of the real world. It aims to create mental models about different areas in which narrative elements such as engagement, conflict, characters, emotionality, meaning, cause-effect relations, and time and space constraints are adapted to convey experiences [1]. A narrative is a vehicle to trigger emotional and cognitive responses to achieve certain serious goals within their context of solicitation. In addition, interaction becomes a matter for decision processes, knowledge creation, communication of nonquantifiable facts, and altering narrative flow to achieve serious contextual goals. Context, course, content, and channel are the four essential components of serious ST. The context is basically the application of circumstances (e.g., medical or psychological problems); the course would be how content evolves in a cause-effect relationship as part of the application context; the content is the actual ideas contained in the narrative; and the channel is the kind of way to communicate stories [1, 2].

With respect to the context, the applications of serious ST in well-being, health, medicine, and psychology are good examples of the multiple possibilities in this field of study [3, 4]. From a scientific point of view, and following Dahlstrom et al., we prefer using the concept of "scientific storytelling" when we apply it in medical investigation [5].

The objectives of our reflection were to propose ST as a tool to offer family support in eating disorders (ED) and to describe the development of the story-based interventions targeted to families (developing communication strategies). It must be noted that ST is a way to communicate (mainly emotional narratives) but not a specific therapy for ED.

With respect to the method, due to the fact that this chapter is based on a future review, which we are developing ("storytelling and health education"), the main data of our reflection are taken from a search using PubMed/MEDLINE and PsycInfo, considering those articles mainly focused on ED and specifically on bulimia nervosa.

Elements	Meaning	Instruments
Narrative	Content (story) Form (discourse)	Time-context Cause-effect Sequence
Perspective	Subjective point of view	Cognition Emotion Encoding-decoding Meaning Memory
Interactivity	Story features	Engagement Modification Narrative flow
Medium	Means of communication	Mediation Channels Forms

Table 1.
Basic components of storytelling.

2. Results

2.1 Storytelling in medicine and psychology

The effectiveness of ST as a communication tool in healthcare has been supported by evidence from several disciplines [6].

Within the healthcare context, ST might be seen as a way of assistance in learning about and managing one's disease or a relative's disease. ST aimed to disease management is based on the fact that each person has his or her own unique experiences living with and managing a disease; the same applies for relatives. Thus, patients and patient relatives' stories are a relevant information source to both patients and families [7].

In this way, storytellers are patients and patients' relatives who suffer together a disease or disorder. By identifying with the storyteller, participants can become invested in the content and be positively influenced by the self-management actions described. Telling stories, emotional stories, is a very good tool to break down cognitive resistance to messages promoting lifestyle and behavioral changes [7] or, many times, to get involved in adequate care and support. Through ST, patients increase their receptivity to the health information contained in the stories as it occurs among patients' families.

In sum, ST is a way to motivate both patients and families [6]. In this regard, ST, as a mechanism for reduction in change resistance, is related to health outcomes [7]; it makes patients and families more inclined to follow strategies that have worked for others (and perhaps they have previously avoided) [8]; it reports mutual benefit (discovery and exploration of new information, practical management strategies and skills, opportunities for adoption of resolutions, etc.) when patients/families exchange their health-related stories [9–11].

When ST is developed in a group format, several authors have reported different benefits [12–15]:

- ST might establish a network of trust and equality among participants, and it would be a way of cohesion among participants.
- ST tends to reduce stigma associated with diseases, and it facilitates the development of relationships among the participants.
- ST can naturally facilitate peer support and enable a support network to form.
- The peer support obtained by means of ST might encourage participants to examine their emotions, problem-solving skills, and goal setting and exchange social support, all of which are core self-management components within health-related contexts.

In summary, ST focuses on the patient's perception of their unique needs and their ability to self-manage their disease and similarly occurs when ST is applied to patients' families. Consequently, ST facilitates both patients and families to develop strategies to manage their illness and suffering, respectively [16].

2.2 Storytelling in chronic diseases

Chronic diseases usually require regular contact between patients/families and therapists. In this particular way, ST could be a good approach for both patient self-management and family management. For this proposal, core principles of

ST, when applied to health contexts, have been reported to be social cognitive and ecological theories of health behavior, caring and healing, and narrative-autobiographical approaches [17–20]. There are two main objectives of ST in health interventions: (a) to get patients/families to reflect the illness experience and (b) to create meaning from it [20].

As Gucciardi et al. have reviewed, health conditions such as diabetes mellitus, cancer, multiple sclerosis, or psychiatric disorders are frequent diseases in which ST has been applied [20]. Sessions of ST are based on informal-spontaneous sharing of stories by means of a nondirective facilitation approach. Sessions do not consist of didactic delivery of information even though "facilitators" (doctor, nurse, dietitian, etc.) can respond to the shared stories and they can also provide information if required. In this context facilitators play a role of equality but not of experts. Finally, ST must have some elemental rules such as trust, respect, empathy, and no judgment [12, 20, 21]. Sometimes it is possible to use "peer facilitators" (e.g., patients' relatives) previously trained as health promoters and, of course, in ST [12].

Sessions of ST applied to chronic diseases tend to be given over 5–15 weeks, with each session lasting 1–2 hours. The environment usually is an open atmosphere, thus giving everyone the opportunity to speak about their experiences. It is convenient to select topics in advance in order that participants prepare the session with the story (or stories) they want to share in the group (e.g., diagnosis experience, course of the disease, family stress linked to the therapeutic aspects, etc.) [22]. The way to share stories is diverse: verbally, by means of action-oriented activities (e.g., cooking, exercising, etc.), using pictures, writing, trough songs, poems, and readings. ST is not a mere colloquium; it is a participant-centered technique of communication where patients and families are encouraged to self-reflect on their personal experiences.

In the context of chronic diseases, ST is not a way of simple catharsis. Telling stories about illness experiences seems to be therapeutic due to its potential to facilitate learning and coping with the disease. As it was noted by Gucciardi et al., ST is a process of unearthing meaning in the lived experience of illness [20]. Telling stories triggers the reflection and understanding of oneself and the disease [23]. The process of ST starts as a single story (my story), and then stories are elaborated by group participants thus becoming a shared experience [21]. Different ages, groups, ethnicities, socioeconomic status, or gender are potential participants of ST applied to health problems. With respect to ideal number of sessions, basing on participants' preferences and bearing in mind the complexity of the self-management of the disease are better. As it was abovementioned, the use of verbal and written formats is the main strategy along with pictures or photographs [20].

The role of narratives has grown in relevance since the 1980s due to the importance of illness experiences. It must be noted that narratives reflect the nature of the chronic disease experiences but also can be a part of it [24].

2.3 Storytelling and eating disorders: families

Traditionally, families are considered to play a key role in the management and treatment of ED. Families do not suffer from an ED, but they live with an ED. In this regard families' stories are a way to create experiences, experiences linked to the emotions which usually accompany a life with an ED.

In the field of ED, families have been associated with relationship alteration within the family, problems between partners, great stress experience, problems to cope successfully, uncertainty regarding recovery progress, parental blaming, etc. [25–30]. ED, as it occurs generally in chronic diseases, might be described as a form of biographical disruption which breaks individual or family-anticipated life paths. As a consequence, narratives lose coherence and meaning and identity becomes lost. The result is a new narrative incoherence which will imply a narrative reconstruction. Stories, ST, will provide new coherences thus giving meaning to ED [31, 32].

Frank [33] considered three narrative types with respect to stories of illness: restitution, chaos, and quest. The first seems to be dominant, and, in sum, it consists of sentences such as "yesterday I was healthy, today I am sick, tomorrow I will be healthy again." On the contrary, chaos narrative is the opposite of restitution, something like "life never will go better again." In this case there is not a narrative coherence to explain the illness. Finally, the quest narrative implies that patients see illness as an opportunity to believe that something is to be gained from the illness experience. Telling stories such as restitution, chaos, or quest narratives has not the same results. Each one shapes experiences. Thus, restitution narratives are usually associated with the fact to pursue, be hopeful, and expect recovery. If the narrative of storytellers shapes their own experiences, the same occurs with regard to the listeners, who, in turn, would also modify their illness experiences [33, 34].

It has been established that ED affect all facets of life and they are a challenging experience for the whole family [34]. It is frequent that parental understandings of illness can remain couched in restitution. Nevertheless, when family members construct ED differently to each other, the consequence is the conflicting narratives and, finally, frustration, anger, and altered communication [34]. Considering the three narratives as suggested by Frank [33], it is possible to observe a process during the therapeutic work in ED (**Figure 1**).

ED are usually chronic disorders, thus being both a challenge and a source of family problems. Within the family system, a process of meaning-making will emerge which is absolutely necessary to cope with the illness. This process is guided by culturally dominant illness narratives as stated by Frank [33].

2.4 Storytelling and eating disorders: patients

When patients with ED are the storytellers, it is possible to distinguish two very different narratives: the discourse of anorectic and bulimic patients [35, 36].

The discourse of patients with anorexia nervosa is built upon three pillars: intensification, circularity, and polarization. This discourse presents a defined reality characterized by excess, conflict, and closing [35].

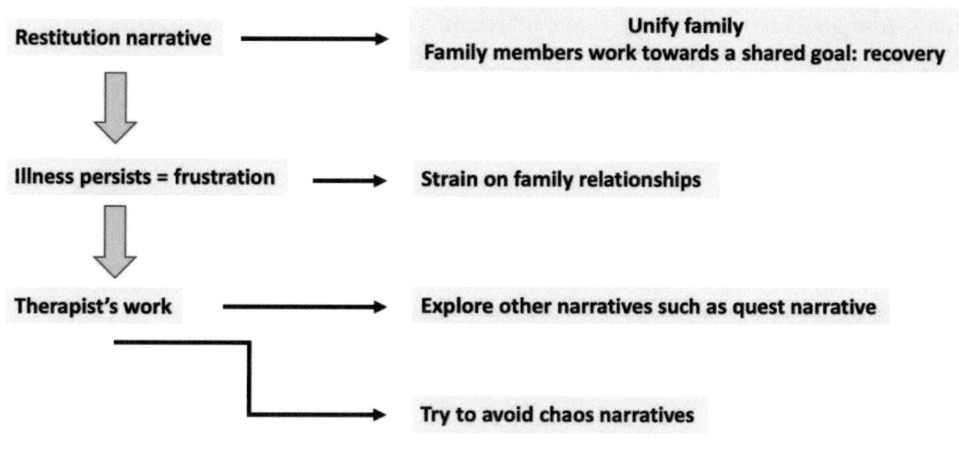

Figure 1.
Therapist working with ED. Adapted from Papathomas et al. [34].

Intensification leads to derealization, thus showing a distorted world with regard to its dimensions. On the one hand, it is a vehicle to express very intense feelings; on the other hand, intensification does not end up with this expressive function since it serves as a strategy to legitimate specific behaviors [35].

The amplified image of reality triggers the alarm; it expresses an obsessive fear to gain weight. Thus, body image is perceived to the limit of bearable, and this seems to justify the obsessive desire to lose weight. Maybe the discourse shows the object: the distorted image acts generating fear, thus becoming a relevant factor which maintains the disorder. The dichotomic vision of reality reinforces anorectic behaviors since that vision implies a fight between contrary parts. The result is an experience of a fragmentary world and a split-off vision with respect to the own conscience. Antithesis, paradoxes, and generally the dialectical approach keep alive and reinforce the awareness of both external and internal confrontation, and, as we have seen, once the conscience is divided between opposing parts, it is always defeated in this war of no one [35, 36].

Circularity, showed linguistically by a high degree of recurrence, creates a net of words which envelops and imprisons. As the water of a fountain reflects the image of Narcissus, anorectic discourse throws an image which locks one inside; that discourse shows a conscience turned on itself, tightly centered and closed on the conflict. From this point of view, anorectic discourse is both an expression and an instrument of the disease. At the same time, that discourse has the keys which might neutralize the disease effects. If the discourse catches and it makes the person sick, it is possible to build another different discourse to create and legitimate a healthy behavior.

Considering positive and negative elements of anorectic discourses, it would be possible to include the analysis of discourse within the whole treatment program. By means of the analysis of recordings and texts, it is possible to think over with a critical point of view about the patients' thinking schemes. Then it would be possible to build an alternative discourse, a new healthy discourse [35].

In the case of bulimia nervosa, as a feature that defines the discourse, its openness from the thematic point of view and also some peculiarities in what refers to the global construction of the discourse should be noted. From the thematic point of view, stories usually show a universe open to others, with a central theme, which is dependent on affection and recognition of others [36].

Following the studies of Márquez [35, 36], considering bulimia nervosa, perhaps the most outstanding feature, along with the fragmentary character of the discourse, is the polyphony: voices of the same person or of the others, real or imagined, that give life to the story, make it rich and complex, and, at all events, show a consciousness inhabited by others, confused with them.

In the syntactic plane, the global organization of the discourse is defined by its scattered character: broken syntax with unfinished structures, suspended utterances, and sudden alterations in rhythm show a specific type of thought which is built on impulses.

Verbalization of experiences, reflection, and reconstruction of memories are emerging to consciousness in a choppy way, in various attempts that are not usually alternatives to saying the same thing (or different ways of approaching a fact), since the first tend to be unsuccessful. Stories are characterized by impulsivity, ruptures, advances, and setbacks, which, in short, express precipitation, lack of a necessary prior time for reflection and planning, lack of containment, and difficulties in adjusting to limits.

Intensification presents facts and sensations as endowed with an extreme force; as a result, reality is constructed with such intensity that it is uncontainable within its natural channels. Thus considered, this resource serves as legitimization of the illness behaviors. Vocalic lengthening and sudden changes in the language rhythm, as well as precipitation and slowing down, also show the presence of emotions that overflow the consciousness, sensations, and affects that are difficult to conduct and finally become not contained.

In short, a broken speech seems to reflect the lack of a coherent internal organizing center, a broken voice, a word that has its justification and its center abroad, as an echo [36].

From a dialogical view of change, it is possible to consider change and resistance to change. Resistance to change derives from the slavery of repeating, which traps the dialogical self. The tension between change (liberty of reborn) and resistance to change (self-determination to repetition) can be also represented as voices discussing and contrasting in the context of a personal arena, in the dynamic of a dialog between parts [37].

2.5 Work with families in eating disorders

It is usual to work with families when an ED patient begins his/her process of treatment. There are two facts which we can observe at this point. Firstly, families tend to express that they never imagined a son or daughter with an ED. Second, it is frequent that families talk about their "fault." Novelty and fault build a recurrent question: Why?

It has been said that healthy relationships are like the tides: they ebb and flow, especially when it comes to verbal interaction. Ebbing and flowing give as a result a balance. But when a family member suffers from an ED, this balance is very hard to maintain. When this occurs, the patient becomes quite self-centered, self-absorbed. Now, relationships as well as dialogs need to be rebalanced. Once an ED affects a family member, many times siblings are victims of that ED since parents focus much more of their time, thoughts, and energy on that affected member. Verbal interactions and relationships are strongly modified. From the point of view of siblings, the patient gets all the love, all the attention, while other members get ignored and overlooked. In order to attract parents' attention, siblings may start some unhealthy behaviors such as rebelling, acting out, etc. [38].

ED often is an enemy of healthy relationships. As an ED develops and progresses, it often takes the place of wholesome relationships that may have once existed in one's life. Typically, as the ED roots within a person, relationships with family members, friends, partners, etc. become strained and gradually altered [39].

Altered relationships within the family tend to create a different discourse. The coherent healthy discourse becomes a broken discourse stained by feelings of doubt, guiltiness, and many times lack of hope. This way a new story emerges. Patients, siblings, parents, partners, etc. have their new particular stories to tell or, sometimes, shut up. During the therapeutic process of ED, there are very different elements that parents refer to as having a great impact on their lives. Examples of these elements would be family unification or disintegration, inability to cope with the disease, inconsiderate comments from significant others, social isolation, and financial impacts, among others. The chronicity of ED causes stress for the family as a unit, by affecting the family's coping mechanisms and the family's relationships with significant others leading to isolation of the family unit [28].

Isolated parents give few insights into the ED experience across the whole family unit. Illness experiences may be analyzed through thematic analyses. Although these content-driven approaches can be useful, they offer scarce for the social construction of the ED experience. Specifically, how personal interpretations of illness are shaped through social and cultural narrative auspices is rarely addressed. It is in this regard how ST would be an appropriate tool to understanding illness. The role of narratives, the role of telling stories, would lead to the deepest personal illness experiences. Narrative therapy for ED is well known since the 1980s. By means of telling stories, therapists work with patients, who create a sort of "anti-anorexia" and "anti-bulimia" stories. These stories aim to depict a separation between the person and the disorder, thus setting up space for patients (and families) to re-envision their relationship with their ED. Patients will create a new personal story "without the ED."

2.6 Bulimia nervosa: patients and families. Dialogical analysis with ST

Along with bulimia nervosa, it has been reported that 61.5% of youth with this ED could be considered to have one or more comorbid disorders (especially mood disorders, anxiety disorders, and personality disorders) [40]. In this particular way, ST might be applied not only in the case of bulimia nervosa but also when comorbidities are present. Thus, using narrative therapy in a group of women with long-course ED with comorbid depression, a reduction in both ED and levels of depression was obtained. It seems necessary to work with different facets: (a) externalize the ED, thus creating distance between herself (patient) and the disorder; (b) explore the person's ED, in which values belong to the patient and which belong to the ED; and (c) develop an alternative story to support the client's sense of self (not just with respect to eating but in other areas of her life); it is not the same "to be" a bulimic patient than "to suffer from bulimia nervosa" [41].

ST is a way of communication, a way to change the discourse, thus contributing to change our mind. Many patients usually say "I can't start again" and "it is impossible to change." But if the patient does not change, the result is the permanence. The same applies to families. Between change and permanence emerges the conflict, and the discourses serve the conflict becoming broken, incoherent. Stories may be based on change and on no change. The consequent discourse is a speech aimed to express the deep desire of change or, on the contrary, the conviction to permanence, the change being impossible. As Marquez stated [35, 36], change vs. non-change is something like an inner dialog between voices, but not only "inner" since external components appear (family, partner, friends, etc.). As stated by Salvini et al. [37], the dialog between voices implies that when one party speaks, the other party is required to be silent. This way, it is common that a dominant discourse emerges (interactional dominance), the dialog being asymmetrical. Therapists must consider this phenomenon because the more symmetrical the dialog is, the more opportunity it provides for mutual influence; the more asymmetrical it is, the more it constrains the exchange of views and experiences. When symptoms are the core part of the discourse and this discourse becomes dominant, patients and families are imprisoned. Following the analysis of Márquez [36], in bulimia nervosa stories are characterized by impulsivity, ruptures, advances, and setbacks, which, in short, express precipitation, lack of a necessary prior time for reflection and planning, lack of containment, and difficulties in adjusting to limits. This style usually leads to a chaos narrative [33].

Based on the study of Hermans et al. [42], Salvini et al. [37] considered the trend toward discursive change during the therapeutic process according to the following four dimensions: (a) interactional dominance, (b) topic dominance, (c) amount of talk, and (d) strategic movements. In a process of scientific ST, it is relevant to analyze linguistic variations probably linked to a transition from a dysfunctional narrative to a new more coherent one. Among a group of bulimic patients (here bulimic storytellers), one of them could be dominant, and the dialog starts being very asymmetrical. With respect to the topics, diets, body image, emotional instability, binge episodes, purging, and other altered behaviors (e.g., self-injuries) are usually highlighted by group members. At the beginning the amount of talk and strategic movements might be summarized as a scarce of true dialog with different attempts to impose one over others. Each member seems to search for a top position in the group, thus polarizing and dominating the other voices [37]. As the sessions go on, a more reciprocal interaction is favored. The topics remain but they are less strong than before. In order to understand these changes, it is necessary to bring here the concept of metaposition, something like a "third voice." This third voice has a reflexive function. Some auxiliary verbs (*I have to be treated*, *I want to get better*, etc.) are contrasted by more verbs which imply personal conditions (*I feel happy*, *I do not like*, etc.). With the progression of the ST process, the preferred tense is the past, thus distinguishing between a previous condition and the current state (*when I binged*, *once I felt frustrated and I used laxatives*, etc.). Step by step a passage from a condition of dysfunctional self-narratives to more organized ones is observed.

As reported by Marquez [36], the discourse may have a relevant role in maintaining the problem, but it is possible to pass from a broken discourse to another healthier one. The discourse reveals psychological profiles as well as interaction styles. In the field of ED, and particularly in bulimia nervosa, working with ST should aim to introduce a "language of change" for both patients and families.

2.7 Topics to listen from bulimic storytellers

Characteristics of bulimia nervosa involve the sufferer bingeing on large amounts of food, during which patients experience feelings of extreme loss of control. Bingeing leaves the patients feeling guilty, disgusted with themselves, and afraid of weight gain. Patients try to compensate for this by vomiting, by exercising, by fasting, by abusing laxatives, or often by some combination of these behaviors. The life of bulimic patients is usually chaotic: dieting, bingeing, purging, fear to weight gain, feeling of being fat, etc. As result, patients have a negative view of themselves which usually leads to avoiding social interactions. Low mood and poor quality of life complete this framework.

In a ST group, some topics will emerge soon:

1. What is bulimia nervosa?
2. Effects of bulimia nervosa in my life (physical, psychological, and social facets)
3. Dieting
4. Is it possible to change my way of thinking?
5. What are thinking errors?
6. Coping with problems and emotions (anxiety, depression, fear, etc.)
7. Body dissatisfaction
8. Assertiveness
9. How is my future?
10. Can I help myself?
11. Bulimia nervosa has many disadvantages for me but has it any advantages?

12. What is a vicious cycle (diet-binge-diet; purge-binge-purge, etc.)?

13. What induces me to binge?

14. What triggers diet-binge-purge?

15. Can I remember what is normal eating?

16. Is this a healthy life?

17. Am I aware of the links among feelings, thoughts, mood, behavior, relationships, etc.?

In ST "emotional meanings" are essential. Patients with ED assign different meanings to their disorder. Those meanings are reflected in their narratives, their illness experiences told in their particular stories. Patients with bulimia nervosa usually have maladaptive thoughts and emotions related to eating habits and body weight. They also have low self-esteem, and they seem to be sure that a well-designed body would be a remedy for their problems of personal insecurity. In this regard, their behaviors aim an idealized body through diets, purging rituals, and often strenuous exercise. The chaos is based on the fact that the desire to lose weight is associated with a personal disorganization. As a result, regulation and control over eating become an attempt to organize and stabilize the chaotic mental state [43]. ST is a good instrument to communicate emotional experiences and a way to access patient's difficulties and internal conflicts. In fact, narratives can be seen as expressions of the self and the living experience for the individual who narrates. The link between individuals and their "bulimic (or anorectic) voice" could explain their ambivalence to change [44–46].

Apart from the abovementioned topics related to the patient's current problems and family-related features, there are different meanings with respect to the onset of the disorder. Low self-esteem, clusters of stressful events, new experiences/difficulties emerged with the disorder, feelings experienced after the onset of the disorder, etc. are usually core parts of the patients' narratives [43].

As other therapeutical approaches, ST aims to produce changes. Patients and families could expect changes to happen such as more dialog, closeness and affection between family members, fewer conflicts between siblings, greater family participation in treatment, more family togetherness, less critical comments, etc. Considering families, the desire to change family dynamics seems to facilitate a healthier environment and consequently a clear improvement in the therapeutic progress. Generally, family emerges as the main source of patients' social support.

3. Discussion and conclusions

ST is a communication tool among human beings with a core aspect which is the emotions. Narratives are a vehicle to trigger emotional and cognitive responses to achieve certain serious goals within their context of solicitation. With respect to the context, the applications of scientific ST in well-being, health, medicine, and psychology are good examples of the multiple possibilities in this field of study. Considering health contexts, storytellers are patients and patients' relatives who suffer together a disease or disorder. In this particular way, ST is a manner to motivate both patients and families, ST being a mechanism for reduction in change resistance, which is usually related to health outcomes. In the context of chronic diseases, ST is not a way of simple catharsis. Telling stories about illness experiences seems to be therapeutic due to its potential to facilitate learning and coping with the disease. ED are usually chronic disorders, thus being both a challenge and a source of family problems. Within the family system, a process of meaning-making will emerge which is absolutely necessary to cope with the illness. This process is guided by culturally dominant illness narratives as stated by Frank, and it was abovementioned [33]. As reported by Marquez [36], the discourse may have a relevant role in maintaining the problem, but it is possible to pass from a broken discourse to another healthier one. The discourse reveals psychological profiles as well as interaction styles. In the field of ED, and particularly in bulimia nervosa, working with ST should aim to introduce a "language of change" for both patients and families. As it was abovementioned, impulsivity, ruptures, advances, and setbacks, which, in short, express precipitation, lack of a necessary prior time for reflection and planning, lack of containment, and difficulties in adjusting to limits, are a cluster which define the interaction between family members and a patient diagnosed with BN. This style usually leads to a chaos in both narrative and relationships (in the case of anorexia nervosa, the circularity—manifested linguistically in the high degree of recurrence—weaves with words a network that envelops and imprisons; the discourse projects an image that encloses the subject within himself; the discourse shows an awareness turned inward, hermetically centered and closed on the conflict, thus affecting a clear dialog with others) [35, 36]. In sum, ST aims to produce changes, in both discourse and relationships. Patients and families could expect changes to happen such as more dialog, closeness and affection between family members, fewer conflicts between siblings, greater family participation in treatment, more family togetherness, less critical comments, etc. Considering families, the desire to change family dynamics seems to facilitate a healthier environment and consequently a clear improvement in the therapeutic progress. Generally, family emerges as the main source of patients' social support.

ST is above and beyond a useful form of communication. ST is not a specific therapy, and its great advantage is to improve the existing therapies by means of a better communication between therapists and patients as well as between family members and patients. With respect to ED, a patient (that is to say a "storyteller") could summarize, in a delightful poem, the process of changing of someone who starts suffering from anorexia or bulimia nervosa (and still is sure to control it) until they reach a point of no return. The capital letter of each verse wants to reflect the inner highness of the affected person.

Due to the original language in which the poem has been written down, we have decided to maintain the Spanish version as well as to translate the poem into English.

I WISHED TO BE...
And I wanted to be waning moon just not to be sun.
And I imagined myself to be fine and delicate rainfall.
And I was a beautiful Caladium with a slender stem.
And I dreamt of being a horse chestnut tree with an upright and leafy trunk.
And I tried to be Artemisa or Apollo.
But I became a goldfinch that could not sing and my colors faded without my knowing why.
And ceased being an Alpha Canis Majoris when my shine dimmed.
When the failed transformation occurred.
All the figures that my mind reflected were slimline.
Until I did not want to be, until I did not think.
Because I was just looking for perfection.

Y QUISE SER...
Y quise ser luna menguante para no ser sol.

Y me imaginé ser lluvia fina y delicada.
Y fui hermosa Caladium de tallo esbelto.
Y soñé ser un castaño de Indias con el tronco erguido y abundante hojas.
Y fingí ser Artemisa o Apolo.
Pero me convertí en un jilguero que no podía cantar y perdí mis colores sin saber la razón.
Y dejé de ser una Alpha Canis Majoris cuando perdí mi brillo.
Cuando sucedió la transformación fallida.
Todas las figuras que mi mente reflejaba eran finas.
Hasta que no quise ser, hasta que no pensé.
Porque solo buscaba la perfección.

Author details

José Vicente Martínez Quiñones[1*], Mar Martínez Gamarra[2]
and Ignacio Jáuregui Lobera[3]

1 Department of Neurosurgery, Mutua de Accidentes de Zaragoza, Zaragoza, Spain

2 Storytelling Spanish Association (ASEST), Spain

3 Department of Molecular Biology and Biochemical Engineering, University of Pablo de Olavide of Seville, Seville, Spain

*Address all correspondence to: jvmartinez@maz.es

References

[1] Lugmayr A, Sutinen E, Suhonen J, Islas Sedano C, Hlavacs H, Suero Montero C. Serious storytelling—A first definition and review. Multimedia Tools and Applications. 2017;**76**:15707-15733

[2] Meadows MS. Pause & Effect: The Art of Interactive Narrative. Indianapolis: Pearson Education, New Riders Press; 2002

[3] Day D. Exercise without failure: Building fitness Apps as narrative game. Model View Culture (Technology, Culture, and Diversity Media) [Online]. 2015. Available from: https://modelviewculture.com/pieces/exercise-without-failure-building-fitness-apps-as-narrative-games

[4] Debra Malina P. Narrative Medicine: Honoring the Stories of Illness. New York: Oxford University Press; 2006

[5] Dahlstrom MF, Scheufele DA. (Escaping) the paradox of scientific storytelling. PLoS Biology. 2018;**16**:e2006720

[6] Hartling L, Scott S, Pandya R, Johnson D, Bishop T, Klassen TP. Storytelling as a communication tool for health consumers: Development of an intervention for parents of children with croup. Stories to communicate health information. BMC Pediatrics. 2010;**10**:64-74

[7] Houston TK, Allison JJ, Sussman M, Horn W, Holt CL, Trobaugh J, et al. Culturally appropriate storytelling to improve blood pressure: A randomized trial. Annals of Internal Medicine. 2011;**154**:77-84

[8] McQueen A, Kreuter MW, Kalesan B, Alcaraz KI. Understanding narrative effects: The impact of breast cancer survivor stories on message processing, attitudes, and beliefs among African American women. Health Psychology. 2011;**30**:674-682

[9] Greenhalgh T, Campbell-Richards D, Vijayaraghavan S, Collard A, Malik F, Griffin M, et al. New models of self-management education for minority ethnic groups: Pilot randomized trial of a story-sharing intervention. Journal of Health Services Research & Policy. 2011;**16**:28-36

[10] Cangelosi PR, Sorrell JM. Storytelling as an educational strategy for older adults with chronic illness. Journal of Psychosocial Nursing and Mental Health Services. 2008;**46**:19-22

[11] Greenhalgh T, Collard A, Begum N. Narrative based medicine: An action research project to develop group education and support for bilingual health advocates and elderly south Asian patients with diabetes. Practical Diabetes International. 2005;**22**:125-129

[12] Greenhalgh T, Collard A, Campbell-Richards D, Vijayaraghavan S, Malik F, Morris J, et al. Storylines of self-management: Narratives of people with diabetes from a multiethnic inner city population. Journal of Health Services Research & Policy. 2011;**16**:37-43

[13] Holm A-K, Lepp M, Ringsberg KC. Dementia: Involving patients in storytelling—A caring intervention. A pilot study. Journal of Clinical Nursing. 2005;**14**(2):256-263

[14] Dale JR, Williams SM, Bowyer V. What is the effect of peer support on diabetes outcomes in adults? A systematic review. Diabetic Medicine. 2012;**29**:1361-1377

[15] Funnell MM. Peer-based behavioural strategies to improve chronic disease self-management and clinical outcomes: Evidence, logistics, evaluation considerations and needs

for future research. Family Practice. 2010;**27**(Suppl 1):i17-i22

[16] Piana N, Maldonato A, Bloise D, Carboni L, Careddu G, Fraticelli E, et al. The narrative-autobiographical approach in the group education of adolescents with diabetes: A qualitative research on its effects. Patient Education and Counseling. 2010;**80**:56-63

[17] Sitvast J. Self-management and representation of reality in photo stories. ANS. Advances in Nursing Science. 2013;**36**:336-350

[18] Evans BC, Crogan NL, Bendel R. Storytelling intervention for patients with cancer: Part 1—Development and implementation. Oncology Nursing Forum. 2008;**35**:257-264

[19] Crogan NL, Evans BC, Bendel R. Storytelling intervention for patients with cancer: Part 2—Pilot testing. Oncology Nursing Forum. 2008;**35**:265-272

[20] Gucciardi E, Jean-Pierre N, Karam G, Sidani S. Designing and delivering facilitated storytelling interventions for chronic disease self-management: A scoping review. BMC Health Services Research. 2016;**16**:249

[21] Koch T, Kralik D. Chronic illness: Reflections on a community-based action research programme. Journal of Advanced Nursing. 2001;**36**:23-31

[22] Greenhalgh T, Collard A, Begum N. Sharing stories: Complex intervention for diabetes education in minority ethnic groups who do not speak English. BMJ. 2005;**330**:628

[23] Sandelowski M. We are the stories we tell: Narrative knowing in nursing practice. Journal of Holistic Nursing. 1994;**12**:23-33

[24] Kleinman A. The Illness Narratives: Suffering, Healing, and the Human Condition. New York: Basic Books; 1988

[25] Gilbert AA, Shaw SM, Notar MK. The impact of eating disorders on family relationships. Eating Disorders. 2000;**8**:331-345

[26] Espina A, De Alda IO, Ortego A. Dyadic adjustment in parents with daughters with an eating disorder. European Eating Disorders Review. 2003;**11**:349-362

[27] Highet N, Thompson M, King RM. The experience of living with a person with an eating disorder: The impact on the careers. Eating Disorders. 2005;**13**:327-344

[28] Hillege SP, Beale B, McMaster R. Impact of eating disorders on family life: Individual parents' stories. Journal of Clinical Nursing. 2006;**15**:1016-1022

[29] Tierney SJ. The treatment of adolescent anorexia: A qualitative research study focusing on the views of parents. Eating Disorders. 2005;**13**:369-379

[30] Vandereycken W. Introduction. Eating Disorders. 2005;**13**:325-326

[31] Bury M. Chronic illness as biographical disruption. Sociology of Health & Illness. 1982;**4**:167-182

[32] Crossley ML. Narrative psychology, trauma and the study of self/identity. Theory & Psychology. 2000;**10**:527-546

[33] Frank AW. The Wounded Storyteller: Body, Illness and Ethics. Chicago, IL: University of Chicago Press; 1995

[34] Papathomas A, Smith B, Lavallee D. Family experiences of living with an eating disorder: A narrative analysis. Journal of Health Psychology. 2015;**20**:313-325

[35] Márquez M. La pena del Espejo. Rasgos lingüísticos propios del discurso de una paciente anoréxica. Trastornos de la Conducta Alimentaria. 2005;**1**:1-29

[36] Márquez M. La palabra de eco. Rasgos lingüísticos propios de una paciente bulímica. Trastornos de la Conducta Alimentaria. 2006;**3**:208-227

[37] Salvini A, Faccio E, Mininni G, Romaioli D, Cipolletta S, Castelnuovo G. Change in psychotherapy: A dialogical analysis single-case study of a patient with bulimia nervosa. Frontiers in Psychology. 2012;**3**:546

[38] Eating Disorder HOPE. Family Involvement in Treatment. 2017. Available from: https://www.eatingdisorderhope.com/treatment-for-eating-disorders/family-role [Accessed: October 27, 2018]

[39] Eating Disorder HOPE. How Eating Disorders Can Affect Relationships. 2017. Available from: https://www.eatingdisorderhope.com/treatment-for-eating-disorders/family-role/how-eating-disorders-can-affect-relationships [Accessed: October 27, 2018]

[40] Pan J. Eating disorders and comorbidity in childhood and adolescence: A comparison between children and adolescents diagnosed exclusively with an eating disorder and those diagnosed with another comorbid condition in addition to the eating disorder. In: Final Outcomes Report. McMaster University; 2009

[41] Narrative Therapy and Eating Disorders: Help or Hype? 2014. Available from: https://www.scienceofeds.org/2014/01/22/narrative-therapy-and-eating-disorders-help-or-hype/ [Accessed: October 29, 2018]

[42] Hermans HJM, Kempen HJG, Van Loon RJP. The dialogical self: Beyond individualism and rationalism. The American Psychologist. 1993;**47**:23-33

[43] Leonidas C, dos Santos MA. Emotional meanings assigned to eating disorders: Narratives of women with anorexia and bulimia nervosa. Annals of Nutritional Disorders & Therapy. 2017;**4**:1040

[44] Granato TM, Aiello-Vaisberg TMJ. Interactive narratives about infant care and its affective-emotional meanings. Psicologia Clínica. 2013;**25**:17-35

[45] Tierney S, Fox JRE. Living with the anorexic voice: A thematic analysis. Psychology and Psychotherapy: Theory, Research and Practice. 2010;**83**:243-254

[46] Hoskins ML. Living research: The experience of researching self, other, and discourse. Journal of Consulting Psychology. 2000;**13**:47-66

Section 4

Clinical Management: Monitoring of Physical and Mental Health and Providing Psychological Therapy

Chapter 9

Reclaiming the Lost Self in the Treatment of Bulimia Nervosa: A Neurobiological Approach to Recovery That Integrates Mind, Brain, and Body

Abigail H. Natenshon

Abstract

The pathology of bulimia nervosa reflects the 'dis-integration' of the structure of the self within the distributed nervous system, resulting in the patient's impaired sense of self and incapacity to sense self-experience. The twenty-first century definition of self as 'an embodied, sensory-based process grounded in kinesthetic experience' not only refutes the long-held myth of mind-body dualism, but also sheds light on the influence of neurobiological factors in disease onset and on how people make recovery changes within psychotherapy. The capacity to create, or reinstate, self-integration is built into the nervous system through the neuroplastic brain's ability to change its structure and function in response to thought, sensation, feeling, and motor activity. The introduction of neurophysiological (sensorimotor) and neurobiological (interpersonal, attachment-based) interventions into mainstream clinical treatment for bulimia nervosa increases exposure to embodied experience, fostering mind, brain, and body connectivity. By stimulating integrative neuronal firing and synaptic activity, top-down and bottom-up transactions enhance acuity in self-sensing, self-perception, and body image coherence, supporting the unification of the disparate self. The current focus of mainstream clinical eating disorder treatment on symptom reduction alone neglects the neurological underpinnings of the disease. This chapter describes a range of treatment options for bulimia nervosa designed to support sustainable changes at the brain level.

Keywords: bulimia nervosa, anorexia nervosa, eating disorders, self-image, body image, self-integration, neurobiology, neurobiological interventions, neurophysiological interventions, trauma resolution, interpersonal neurobiology, Feldenkrais Method, sensorimotor interventions, embodied self, disorganized attachment, mind-brain-body connections, vertical integration

1. Introduction

Bulimia nervosa (BN), described as "an ominous variant of anorexia nervosa" (AN) [1], is a disorder of the brain, the distributed nervous system, and the pathological 'dis-integration' of the core self, all indicators of mind, brain, and body disconnection. Scientists propose that somatic, autonomic, and visceral information is aberrantly processed in people who are vulnerable to developing AN and/or BN [2]. Engaging the distributed nervous system in the treatment of BN through adjunctive interventions that combine top-down and bottom-up neurophysiological mechanisms, and/or through the psychobiological attachment bond of emotional communication and interactive regulation between the patient and therapist, heals neurobiological aberrations at their source by accessing the roots of these disorders, which are embedded in neurobiological dysfunction. By capturing images of the neuroplastic brain as it changes in real time, modern brain-scanning technology reveals that harnessing body-based movement and sensory experience in conjunction with psychotherapy facilitates the neurological convergence of the mind, brain, and body, which fosters the integration of the structure of the healthy self. The current focus of mainstream conventional BN treatment, however, is on the psychological and environmental origins of the disorder, neglecting the neurological underpinnings of disease. Scientific evidence points to the need to expand the parameters of the treatment field to promote the neurobiological reintegration of the recovering bulimic patient's healthy self through treatment modalities that sustain changes at the brain level. Recruiting brain circuitry enhances and promotes the integration of the nervous system. "It is around the concept of the core self that psychology crosses paths with the brain and body" [3].

The etiology of neurobiological disturbances leading to ED onset stems from genetic, metabolic, and other biological factors, in conjunction with ever-changing internal forces and external circumstances, compounded by the influence of co-occurring diagnoses. BN symptomatology, marked by behavioral excess and impulsivity, anesthetizes or otherwise reorganizes the patient's affective and internal states. Symptoms typically include bingeing, self-induced vomiting, fasting, food restriction, promiscuity, self mutilation, stealing, compulsive shopping, compulsive exercise, abuse of substances including alcohol, laxatives, diuretics, and/or diet pills, erratic sleep patterns, and the compulsion to prepare food for others.

Alike in their neurobiological underpinnings, AN and BN patients share disturbances in their capacity to experience the sensation of hunger, and typically relieve distress through symptomatic behaviors that create a sense of control over internal chaos and frightening emotions. Diagnostic distinctions between BN and AN are never well delineated. A subgroup of anorexic patients purges; a subgroup of bulimic patients restricts food in the presence, or absence, of bingeing and/or purging. Although abnormally low body weight is an exclusion for the diagnosis of BN, some 25–30% of individuals with BN have a prior history of AN [4]. The greatest levels of psychopathology are present in patients whose diagnoses cross over from AN to BN, or from BN to AN [5], a phenomenon seen in restricting-type AN patients who attempt to eat normally, then fearing the loss of self-control leading to weight gain, couple restrictive eating behaviors with episodes of bingeing and purging; and in BN patients who stop purging, then in an effort to maintain thinness, turn to food restriction or excessive exercise. The binge-purging behaviors of BN lead to a less favorable prognosis than that of restricting-type AN, as dangerous habit-forming and self-perpetuating behaviors lead to potassium depletion and other physical complications [1]. Fifty to eighty percent of the variance in AN and BN liability can be accounted for by genetic factors [2].

This chapter discusses a range of neurophysiological and neurobiological treatment interventions, which, when used as adjuncts to current traditional psychotherapeutic interventions, hold the potential to improve the efficacy and sustainability of ED healing. Because women are more likely than men to perceive their bodies negatively [6], the chapter's focus is on women, with particular attention, through case examples, to those whom I have treated through my practice of psychotherapy.

My concomitant training as a practitioner of the Feldenkrais Method of Somatic Education© has offered me powerful insights into the usefulness of neurophysiological interventions in facilitating healthy self- and body image development. I share some of these insights with readers through anecdotal case examples from my own practice, in conjunction with mindful meditation techniques and Feldenkrais interventions.

2. The neurobiology of AN and BN

"The brains of individuals who exhibit eating ED pathology are 'wired' differently [from non-ED brains], creating the need to define diagnosis by aberrations in brain circuitry and physiology, and then provide treatments aimed at correcting or ameliorating the aberrant circuitry" [7]. Neurocognitive and brain imaging studies suggest that ED patients have impaired neural systems implicated in executive functions, visuospatial processes, self-image perception, emotional regulation and reward processing [8]. "New brain-imaging technology provides insights into ventral and dorsal neural circuit dysfunction—perhaps related to altered serotonin and dopamine metabolism—that contributes to the puzzling symptoms found in people with eating disorders. For example, altered insula activity could explain interoceptive dysfunction, and altered striatal activity might shed light on altered reward modulation in people with AN" [2]. Patients with AN have shown overlapping brain networks involved in reward and behavioral compulsivity [9]. The AN individual's trait toward an imbalance between serotonin and dopamine pathways may play a role in an altered interaction between ventral (limbic) neurocircuits, which are important for identifying the emotional significance of stimuli and for generating an affective response to these stimuli, and dorsal (cognitive) neurocircuits that modulate selective attention, planning and effortful regulation of affective states [2]. Dopamine-related reward circuitry, pathways that modulate the drive to eat, showed reduced activation in this network in BN women; the greater the frequency of binge-purge episodes, the less responsive was the brain [10].

Starvation and emaciation have profound effects on the functioning of the brain and other organ systems, causing neurochemical disturbances that could exaggerate premorbidity, giving rise to symptoms that maintain or accelerate the disease process. Restrictive eating behaviors have been shown to create adverse structural changes in brain regions that are part of the reward circuitry, and also cause shrinkage in the overall size of the brain, including both gray and white matter [8]. Studies of patients with AN show widespread gray matter decreases in the neocortex and in areas linked to emotion regulation and reward, such as the anterior cingulate, orbitofrontal cortex, insular cortex, hippocampus/parahippocampus, amygdala and striatum; studies also report gray matter increases in neocortical and limbic regions. Such volume alterations may, or may not, normalize following ED recovery, dependent upon the severity and endurance of pathology [8]. Puberty may play an active role in major reorganization of white matter during adolescence and early adulthood [8], and activation of a genetic predisposition for ED symptoms. Menarche is associated with a rapid change in body composition and neuropeptides modulating metabolism. It has been surmised that the rise in estrogen levels in pubescent females could affect neuromodulatory systems such as serotonin or neuropeptides that affect feeding, emotionality, and other behaviors [2].

Multiple and distributed brain regions have been implicated in the psychopathology of AN, implying a dysfunction of interregional brain connectivity [8]. A study of structural connectivity suggests that people with AN may have impaired "wiring" between parts of the brain that are involved in the formulation of insight

[9]. An example is brain network connective abnormalities that exist within the caudal anterior cingulate and the posterior cingulate, regions crucial for insight, error detection, conflict monitoring, and self-reflection. One study showed that in AN patients, these regions are poorly connected with the rest of the brain, as compared to healthy participants [9].

Body image distortion may be coded in parietal, frontal, and cingulate regions that assign motivational relevance to sensory events [4]. The parietal cortex mediates perceptions of the body and its activity in physical space. "Recent research extends this concept to suggest that the parietal lobe contributes to the experience of the patient being an 'agent' of her own actions. The well-known distortion of body image in individuals with AN may suggest abnormalities of circuits through the postulated 'self' networks" [4]. Reindl [11] describes BN as a disorder of the self, involving the patient's neurological incapacity to sense self-experience. Bulimic women in recovery report increasing accuracy in "sensing their own voice, sensing that they matter as human beings, sensing what to expect within the change process, and sensing their own curiosity [rather than fear] about their subjective experience" (in [11], pp. 281–282).

> *After engaging in treatment for BN, Emma began to develop a sense that her life matters, and that she has needs that deserve to be recognized by others. Feeling safer and stronger now, through her newly emerging sense of self, in response to her controlling husband's insistence that she terminate treatment, she replied, "Therapy has become my world now. It is nothing that I plan to stop soon."*

3. Factors contributing to BN onset: genetics loads the gun; the environment pulls the trigger

A child with a genetic susceptibility to develop addictions, clinical eating disorders, depression and/or anxiety, having been exposed to the neurobiological effects of chronic early parent/child attachment disturbances, becomes vulnerable to the onset of AN or BN in later life. "The early years of a child's life are the most pivotal time for ground floor development of identity and self-image. Failure of caregivers' appropriate responses to a child's needs deprives the developing child of the essential groundwork for acquiring her own body identity, with a discriminating perceptual and conceptual awareness of her own functions" (in [12], p. 57).

> *Emma, having been bulimic for many decades, reports that when, as an adult, she was 100 pounds overweight, she never experienced herself as being "a fat person." Following bariatric surgery, at a normal weight, she was unable to perceive herself as having become thinner, which motivated her to begin restricting her caloric intake. "In an exercise class one day," she reported, "I caught a glimpse of myself in the mirror and was surprised.... "Who is that person?" I thought. "Could that really be me?"*

The awareness of oneself as a separate individual evolves only through *experiences* and *continuous interaction* with one's environment (in [12], p. 57). "Attuned, empathic responses from caregivers to the child's basic narcissistic needs are experienced by the child as part of the self, and are essential for the development of a healthy self-structure. For example, the caregiver needs to soothe when the child needs calming, enliven when the child needs stimulation, affirm when the child needs coherence" (in [11], p. 39). "When the child's narcissistic needs are disregarded, she becomes vulnerable to an experience of fragmentation and depletion (in [11], p. 39). "By not listening and responding appropriately to a child's needs, parents deprive the child of the opportunity to learn how to listen and respond appropriately to *herself*" (in [11], p. 39). The child whose care-giver uses food as a reward for compliant behavior, or withholds it as punishment, will grow up confused and unable to differentiate her various needs, feeling helpless in controlling her biological urges and emotional impulses (in [12], p. 57). Non-secure relational attachment through neglect or abuse by caregivers in a child's early experience interrupts the production of integrative neuronal fibers within the integrative regions of the brain, which include the amygdala, hippocampus, and prefrontal cortex, where the capacity for self-regulation is located [13].

When a child's genuine needs and affects are consistently met with chronologically inadequate empathy by caregivers, these "needs and affects become disavowed, repressed, or split off from the total self-structure" within the nervous system (in [11], p. 35). The individual's emotional development, once derailed, is unavailable to be integrated into the adult personality (in [11], p. 36). The child not only fails to internalize a healthy self-structure, but eventually creates a new self-system with the split-off aspects of the self. If the individual later begins to experiment with bulimic behaviors, the biochemical effects of the binge-purge cycle create an altered state, reinforcing the already existing split in the psyche, and further organizing the dissociated needs into a 'bulimic self.' Essentially, the BN individual invents a system by which disordered eating patterns, rather than people, are used to meet self-object needs (in [11], p. 36).

Without adequate self-structure, the child experiences herself as ineffective in communicating her internal states to others. Feeling worthless and unlovable contributes to the development of a deep sense of shame. Repeated shame-inducing interpersonal experiences in childhood, once internalized, become an enduring, core sense of shame, spreading throughout the self, shaping one's emerging identity. Contained within the experience of shame is the piercing awareness of one's self as fundamentally deficient, in some vital way, as a human being (in [11], p. 15).

Tess has struggled with BN for decades. Throughout her childhood, she endured her mother's on-going judgment and criticism about her weight. Disagreeing with the pediatrician, Tess' mother considered her daughter "fat," and forbade her to eat the sweet and savory treats offered to her brothers. Tess experienced a searing sense of shame each time her mother warned her not to "let food cross her lips," or forced her to cross her legs to prove that she hadn't yet become too fat to do so. Tess reported, "She informed me in the third grade that when I reached grade five, I could attend Weight Watchers meetings." Decades later, Tess explained, "Having food in my stomach still opens the floodgates of shame and embarrassment from my childhood, bringing me back to those immense feelings of inadequacy and incompetency. My greatest shame of all was in how unworthy I felt to be my mother's child." Early childhood feelings of helplessness and confusion reinforced Tess' continued inability to control her urges and impulses and differentiate her needs and desires well into her adult years.

Dysfunctional family systems of BN individuals tend to generate greater mutual neglect, rejection, and blame, and less understanding, nurturance, and support than do more functional families. The obsessions and compulsions connected to BN symptoms provide the individual a protective shield against disintegration and internal collapse within the hostile and critical family environment, as well as a sense of internal coherence that calms, numbs, or stimulates, as needed.

Tess reports spending much of her childhood in her closet, hidden and isolated, shut off from her family's chaotic world. "I felt invisible and safe there, muffling the sounds of my family's screaming and arguing, protecting myself from having to witness my father physically abusing my brothers." Decades later, at the start of treatment, Tess was still seeking refuge from shame and disgrace behind closed (bathroom) doors now, hiding her purging behaviors from her husband and children. "My feelings of disgrace about needing to soothe myself by purging food and feelings have haunted, and followed me, throughout my life."

The quality of early caregiving "not only affects the child's subjective experience in the moment, but also influences the on-going development of her brain, effecting how her brain will process experience in the future" (in [11], p. 49).

3.1 BN onset typically postdates childhood

Setting the neurological stage for the onset of BN in later life, early childhood abuse or neglect impairs the structure of the self within the nervous system. The abused or neglected young child does not yet have the emotional, developmental, or environmental wherewithal to engage in compensatory behaviors, such as purging, substance abuse, or excessive exercise, all characteristic of BN pathology. BN onset usually emerges in later years, during adolescence or young adulthood, continuing into later years and decades if untreated and unresolved. Early life experiences that influence the mental and emotional characteristics of the child alter the anatomic, physiologic, and metabolic [neurobiological] characteristics of the adult [12]. As adults, BN individuals who have undergone early attachment disorganization impose various forms of abuse and degradation upon themselves, reminiscent of those sustained in childhood.

Women with BN avoid turning inwards to sense their needs, desires, feelings and aggressive strivings, for fear of encountering annihilating disgrace and inadequacy, compounded by guilt.

Emma considered engagement in any form of self-care as equivalent to "intolerable selfishness." Incapable of sensing her own needs and self-experience at the start of treatment, Emma could not discern whether her expressions of kindness or consideration towards her friends were based on honest feelings, or if they were merely "self-serving manipulations," designed to insure the friendship of women whose love and favor she felt she did not deserve.

Profoundly disconnected from their subjective psychic and physical experience, BN individuals feel the need to rely on externally based, rather than internally sensed, gauges to guide their actions.

Emma said, "Because my judgment about everything is so poor, and my thoughts and opinions are never right or acceptable, I have had to rely on my husband to know what is right for the two of us. For close to 25 years of marriage, I have had to 'suck it up,' accepting what he likes, and doing what he wants.... I am also well aware that if I were ever to cross him, the emotional costs for me would be high."

As a disorder of the self, BN is characterized by the individual's diminished self-control, self-regulation, self-attunement, self-trust, self-agency, self-reliance, self-perception, self-sensing and self-worth. As an escape from consciousness of the self, and in response to deficits in self-structure and self-regulatory capacities, BN behaviors separate [dissociate] the patient from her painful thoughts and feelings. "Dissociation implies that two or more mental processes or contents are not associated or integrated, with the result that consciousness, memory, identity, and perception are to some extent disconnected and not experienced as a whole" (in [11], pp. 15, 34).

> *Despite Tess' substantive progress in her BN recovery, her husband's "surprise attack" over dinner one night felt to her like an undeserved and highly demeaning insult. Tess described her immediate, entirely bodily-centered reaction; "I completely shut-down. I went into "blackout mode," totally disconnecting from him, my feelings, and my self. I purged my dinner, along with my feelings, which I had been completely unable to identify till I felt my stomach completely empty. It was only after the violence of that event that I became calm enough to realize what a fool I'd been for believing that he values me and the person that I am becoming."*

Tess had little access to her thinking brain until after her stomach had had its way with her, a phenomenon demonstrating a rift in the fabric of her self-structure. Nervous system re-integration (i.e., healing) takes place over time and through therapeutic life experience, particularly when long-term dysfunction has been ingrained in neuronal development. Significantly however, Tess' capacity to bring her left-brain online in the face of traumatic memory was becoming appreciably more rapid and consistent. In starting to put words to her feelings, she had begun to create a coherent narrative that contained more constructive options for problem resolution.

4. Treating the human nervous system reintegrates mind, brain, and body

In describing how nervous system interconnections occur, Daniel Siegel defines the brain as "a *self*-organizing emergent process of electrochemical energy exchange between brain and body, and with other individuals" [14] and the human mind as "a relational and embodied process that regulates the flow of energy and information" [15]. The roots of the embodied mind exist in the somatic reality of the body. When the dynamic interaction between body and brain is activated, the regulation of energy and information flow happens "not only in the circuits and synapses of the skull-based brain, but also within the body, in the distributed nervous system" (in [15], p. 54). Feedback from sensory receptors throughout the body creates and re-creates the embodied self. Patients access the embodied self through sensing it, in response to self-experience. "The body, as represented in the brain by a map, may constitute the indispensable form of reference for the neural processes that we experience as the mind" [3].

Norman Doidge explains how it all works. "We tend to think of learning as having internal origins within the cranial brain in thoughts, ideas and feelings (top down, and 'from the inside out'). But this is only partly the case. Brain-changing electrical movements also originate in externalized behaviors, through experience and behaviors, affecting the brain 'from the outside in,' addressing different regions [16]. The brain is a feedback loop system, seeking balance and coherence through its own integration in order to achieve and maintain homeostasis [15]. It changes its structure and function with each different activity it performs, continually perfecting its circuits so as to be better suited to any task at hand [17]. "All experience encompassing thought, sensation, feeling, and behavior, be it conscious or unconscious, is embedded in neurons, with neuroplastic change occurring through the movement of ions in and out of brain membranes. Set off by a dynamic flow of electrochemical energy that creates electrical signals and patterns inside neurons, the movement of ions increases the density of brain circuitry within and between various regions of the brain where healing change occurs. Where attention goes, neural firing occurs, and where neurons fire, new connections can be made" (in [16], p. 18).

Contained within the nervous system and grounded in perception and kinesthetic experience, body image and self-image are "virtually interchangeable within the brain, each having mental and neurophysiological components embedded in neurons. There is no valid distinction to be made between the "mind-self" and the "embodied self" (in [18], p. 18). Body image [and self image] change from action to action, built from sensory and psychic experiences that are constantly being integrated in the central nervous system (in [12], p. 87). "It is through self-awareness/consciousness of body and brain that we clarify self-image and body image, experiencing both as an inseparable whole. The unity of body and mind is an objective reality. All feelings and emotions have motoric antecedents initiated within the body" [19]. In other words, "emotions themselves are body phenomena," [20] with the body experiencing emotions first, prior to the mental awareness of feelings. Experiencing emotions is therefore synonymous with experiencing body and brain changes; the development of self-regulation becomes synonymous with regulating changes in both the body and the brain. In BN individuals who have experienced trauma, the brain, which interprets the traumatic event as still happening, will become calmed only following the calming of the body, which under the right circumstances, becomes capable of healing itself, along with emotional wounds.

5. Defining mental health as nervous system integration

The best predictor of positive mental health is nervous system integration [14]. The mind seeks to achieve mental health through "self-organization, optimizing function by linking differentiated parts of the [nervous] system in the quest for harmony, flexibility, resiliency, adaptability, stability, coherence and energy... otherwise known as integration" [15]. In recognizing the body as the first responder to emotional stimuli, the task at hand in healing BN patients is to differentiate emotions from physiological activation. Cognitive self-regulation of emotional responses to aversive events is essential for mental and physical health. Emotion regulation involves a coherent relationship with the self... in other words, the effective, integrative communication between body, mind, and feelings [21]. "A prerequisite for successful emotion regulation is the awareness of emotional states, which in turn is associated with the awareness of bodily signals, or interoceptive awareness" [22]. "The human body needs to sense, process, and integrate different bodily signals in the premotor, temporoparietal, posterior parietal, and extrastriate cortices, in order to achieve self-identification, self-location, and body-part ownership" [23]. "Stimulating interoceptive sensing of body signals facilitates the differentiation of emotions from the physiological component of emotional experience, promoting self-regulation," [22] a process central to healing sub-clinical, as well as clinical, eating disorders and dysfunctions of all kinds. A direct correlation exists between a full and integrative ED recovery, and the achievement of central nervous system integration within the treatment process. A survey of recovered ED patients identified "dimensions of psychological self-adaptability and resilience *within a complete and integrative* mental health model" as the fundamental criteria for having achieved recovery success [24]. In retrospect, it is not unusual for recovered ED individuals to express appreciation and gratitude for having experienced the twice-difficult ordeal of taking on the life-threatening challenges of illness, followed by the life-enhancing challenges of the psychotherapeutic healing process.

6. Integrative disorders require integrative approaches to treatment

Currently, conventional psychosocial, behavioral and pharmacological treatment interventions for adults with BN and AN have been shown to have limited efficacy [25]. Hilde Bruch, a pioneer in the field of ED treatment, contends that unsatisfactory treatment results are related to inadequate conceptualizations of the underlying problems (deficits in self-perception and inner controls) (in [12], pp. 378–379). By re-defining the self as "an embodied, sensory-based process grounded in kinesthetic experience" [15], twenty-first century brain research and the field of interpersonal neurobiology have opened new possibilities for the treatment of the impaired BN self, shedding light on *how* people make changes within the context of psychotherapy. In healing the self, therapeutic interventions that access the embodied brain (sensory receptors embedded within, and distributed throughout the body), together with the cranial-based thinking brain, best address the broader neurobiological issues that underlie the inception and maintenance of eating disorders.

"Greater attention to improving the efficacy of existing ED treatment methodologies is critical, given the increasing prevalence of ED, the high risk of relapse, the effects of concurrent psychopathology, the high cost of care, and the greatest mortality rate of all the mental health disorders, which is one in ten patients [25]. Treatment outcome studies for cognitive-behavioral therapy (CBT), currently considered 'best practice' for the treatment of BN, reveal that only 50% of BN subjects stop bingeing and purging even under the very best conditions" [25]. Neurobiological solutions for the impairment of self-structure exist within the patient's learned capacity to sense self-experience, a process defined as "attunement to one's subjective felt experience... a 'felt sense,' being both psychic and bodily, beginning with the body and occurring in the zone between the conscious and the unconscious. Turning inward to consult this 'border zone' leads to the capacity to trust in one's subjective experience, from which emotions, cognitions and memories arise, fostering deep therapeutic changes" (in [11], p. 12), and access to an ever deeper and more complex sense of self" (in [11], p. 99).

Clinicians enhance the patient's capacity to integrate self-based consciousness through focusing on body-felt sensations connected to the emotions and underlying issues that bring her to treatment [15].

> *At one point during a therapy session, I felt I had lost connection with Emma, noticing her eyes beginning to divert from mine, and her increasing discomfort. "What are you feeling right now?" I inquired. Closing her eyes and grimacing, she sat forward on the couch and reported that what we were discussing was making her feel uncomfortable. In response to my inquiry about where in her body she might be sensing this discomfort, Emma replied that it was "in her stomach" and that she was starting to feel nauseated. Previously, she had relinquished responsibility for her purging, blaming her stomach for "dictating" when and where purging would occur. Now she would choose to take responsibility for preventing this from happening. "Why don't we spend a few minutes breathing together," I suggested. The experience altered her emotional state. At this point, with her left-brain on board she began to use words to communicate her feelings of distress, and was relieved to report that her stomach agitation was subsiding. The first stirrings of Emma's feelings of relief, accomplishment, and self-agency were the result of her refusal to succumb to an interruption in the flow of that session by engaging in BN behaviors.*

"The more completely a patient accesses and uses her entire muscular apparatus, the more the brain will become activated, with the activated regions further stimulating adjacent areas," [26] increasing exposure to self-experience and the patient's potential to sense it (in [11], p. 162).

Providing new ways "to pay attention within the integration of consciousness enables the client with an open and receptive mind to catalyze the integration of new combinations of previously isolated segments of his or her mental reality"

[27]. Studies show that "patients who have been trained to attend to bodily information display greater coherence between subjective experience and visceral responses during emotional episodes" [28]. Because the self, the brain, the mind, and the body are integrated entities, none will heal effectively and sustainably apart from the others.

7. Neurophysiological interventions integrate mind, brain, body, and self

Logic will not change emotion, but body movement will [13]. Straddling verbal and non-verbal input, and "breaking through to feeling," (in [12], p. 46) neurophysiological interventions use the body to create changes in the brain, and the brain to create changes in the body, through top-down and bottom-up processing. Top-down brain processing refers to perception driven by cognition, including mechanisms initiated via mental processing at the level of the cerebral cortex [29, 30]. "Bottom-up brain processing refers to the processing of sensory information as it is coming in [29]. Bottom-up mechanisms are initiated by stimulation of various somato-, viscero-, and chemo-sensory receptors that influence central neural processing and mental activities via ascending pathways from the periphery to the brainstem and cerebral cortex. All mind-body therapies actually involve a combination of top-down and bottom-up mechanisms, creating 'vertical' integration, which brings the emotional and thinking brain online together [30]. Bidirectional autonomic and neuroendocrine pathways serve as mind-body pathways between the central nervous system and the periphery, facilitating the expression of affective, autonomic, hormonal, and immune responses, enhancing mental and physiological functioning [30].

As adjuncts to traditional ED treatment techniques, top-down and bottom-up "neurophysiological interventions have been shown to diminish symptoms associated with ED" [31], contradicting feelings of helplessness and fear, and facilitating a sense of empowerment [13].

> *During her assessment session, it became apparent that Suellyn, who had struggled with BN and major depression for several years, had undergone significant trauma in her past. At 22, she described herself as "always suicidal, feeling way too fat, and frequently being too depressed to get out of bed." She refused to speak of events in her past, believing that doing so would "send her back under the covers." Her mother had recently forced here to leave her home, friends and job, to live temporarily with her father in another state. Seeking a breakthrough to a window of communication, I invited her to consider deep breathing together with me, further awakening her body-felt sensibility through spine twisting, accompanied by differentiated eye movements. Her initial response to the movement was to feel "totally disconnected" from her body, and from me. After about 5 minutes of movement in her chair, she reported, "I am here now," a reality that had become clearly apparent in her eyes and facial expression. She left the session in an elevated mood, planning to return soon.*

Bottom-up interventions have been shown to be more successful in addressing "the repetitive, unbidden, physical sensations, and movement inhibitions, than are top-down interventions" [34]. Providing a non-threatening way to intercept trauma-based memory pathways, bodily-based movement reverses the sensorimotor intrusions of unresolved trauma by conveying to the patients that sensations come and go, leading to their acceptance, and to feeling safer [13].

In the next section, I discuss two types of interventions through which nervous system re-integration fosters the repair of the impaired self. The first involves *neurophysiological* sensorimotor bodily-based movement *with mindful attention and intention*, (differentiating it from rote, 'mindless' bodily exercise). Examples include the Feldenkrais Method, trauma-informed yoga and EMDR. The second is *neurobiological* in nature, repairing the impaired self within a top-down, bottom-up attachment theory model that harnesses the power of empathy within the interpersonal psychotherapeutic connection through empathic resonance. Within this interpersonal neurobiological model, "the top-down process involves cognitive perspective taking, while the bottom-up process, achieved through neuronal mirroring representation systems, plays a key role in the direct sharing of the emotional state of the other" [32]. Rapid Resolution Therapy (RRT) represents a form of neurobiological intervention, specifically designed to achieve the resolution of trauma. Within the context of a trusting relationship, the therapist's focus during RRT is on a neurolinguistic use of oneself within the therapeutic relationship, with the intention of facilitating the patient's self-integration by turning traumatic memories into strengths and resources through memory consolidation [33].

7.1 Sensorimotor psychotherapy

Sensorimotor treatment is a movement-based neurophysiological intervention that combines cognitive and somatic techniques to address physical symptoms of a dissociative nature. Sensorimotor interventions foster healing through the organic, non-reductionist process of 'embodied learning,' which, rather than separating the organism into its anatomical parts, joins those parts into one continuous feedback loop [19]. "In sensorimotor psychotherapy, top-down, cortically mediated functions are harnessed to observe and facilitate sensorimotor processing where patients observe and report the interplay of physical sensation, movements, and impulses, noticing internal reactions as they try out new physical actions. Patients also learn to observe the effects of their thoughts and emotions on their body, recognizing which parts of the body respond to the impact of a particular thought, and/or how the body organizes a particular emotion. Meaning-making emerges from such observation, [resulting in] subsequent transformation of habitual response tendencies" [34]. The process of embodied learning has been shown to "repair and re-integrate perceptual-sensory dysfunction, increase interoceptive attention and/or proprioceptive awareness (the internal awareness of body parts), and produce a more accurate body perception and undistorted body representation" [35]. "Combining sensorimotor bottom-up processes with top-down processes activates the dynamic state of body and brain interaction where the regulation of energy and information flow happens within the circuits and synapses of the skull-based brain, within the body through the distributed nervous system, [and between the brains of two people in the context of a mindful relationship].... all are unifying elements of a disparate self" (in [15], p. 54).

7.1.1 The Feldenkrais Method of Somatic Education© integrates the self and body image coherence

Sensory stimuli are closer to our unconscious, subconscious, or autonomous functioning than to any of our conscious understanding: "Words can obscure intentions; kinesthetic truth gets right to our core" [19]. The Feldenkrais Method promotes self-integration by fostering conscious reconnection with one's unconscious sensorimotor repertoire through expanding the movement repertoire [17]. Directed mindful attention brings previously unfamiliar body parts systematically into awareness, moving the individual and brain toward integration, and offering a concrete means by which to change one's state of being. During or following movement sequences, the essentially non-verbal movement experience might be enhanced through open-ended, insightful verbal cueing that prompts the sensing of self-experience by promoting a coherent narrative within the process, i.e., "Do you sense a place in your body that feels more comfortable and safe...more unfamiliar and unsafe? What is it like for you to explore yet unknown parts of your body and self?"

Within the Feldenkrais sensorimotor movement experience, the clarification of self-image requires the patient's felt-sense during the action, through focused attention on self-awareness (self consciousness), variation (change and novelty), differentiation (the capacity to sense and create differences,) and integration (the capacity to bring the learning to a meaningful coherence). The differentiation and integration of coherent movement coordination provides the critical interface between brain and body, allowing global mapping to be maintained, refreshed and altered by continual motor activity and rehearsal" [3]. Differentiation of the smallest possible sensory distinctions between movements while paying close attention to injured or distorted body parts allows people to subjectively experience these parts through larger, more accurate and refined brain maps (in [18], p. 171).

During Feldenkrais Awareness through Movement [ATM] group classes, conducted on yoga mats, the floor becomes an invaluable feedback system. The practitioner guides participants through scripted sequential movements, facilitating their introspective sensing of self-experience. Feldenkrais Method practice has, through the past eight decades, become increasingly accessible worldwide. It has also become available free-of-charge through easy-to-follow 5 to 20 minute Awareness through Movement© UTube demonstrations presented by expert Feldenkrais practitioners who bring adjunctive sensorimotor movement interventions directly into the clinical treatment office, and/or into patients' homes for independent practice. The Feldenkrais Functional Integration [FI] technique offers hands-on, gentle, pleasurable body movement, promoting self-integration through movement provided through human touch. While the patient lies on the treatment table, the practitioner's nervous system, in connection with the patient's nervous system, imparts sensory information directly to the patient's brain through the patient's embodied sensory receptors. The following examples illustrate the efficacy of the Feldenkrais Method's Awareness through Movement© and Functional Integration© modes as adjuncts to traditional mainstream treatment for patients in recovery from BN.

7.1.1.1 Feldenkrais Awareness through Movement [ATM] as part of mainstream BN practice

> *Marion, a 43-year-old bulimic woman who grew up in a chaotic, dysfunctional family, was diagnosed with BN restricting-type, bi-polar disorder, dissociation, and self-mutilation after having been gang raped by her brother and his friends when she was 16. For close to two decades, she had been treated in hospital programs for BN and post-traumatic stress disorder (PTSD) before joining an outpatient movement-based ED support/therapy group for adults with clinical ED, which I facilitated. Each group session included a guided Feldenkrais Awareness through Movement© lesson, followed by participants processing their movement experience as it relates to relevant therapeutic issues. Though in a food-restrictive phase of her disorder, attunement to her inner bodily experience during group movement sessions led Marion to report that after group sessions, she would go to a grocery store and bring home "a four course dinner." "While eating, I visualize the food as it enters my body as no longer being 'the enemy.' I imagine it traveling around and throughout my entire body, nourishing and giving life to all my cells and tissues." In reconnecting with parts of herself that had previously seemed unsafe, she experienced her self as becoming increasingly "whole." In individual psychotherapy, she began to access*

> *feelings and issues that she ordinarily would not have felt comfortable facing or disclosing. Describing her Feldenkrais experience, she said, "I know I am safe. I know where I am in my body, and I know that I am learning to know myself better. This work makes me feel that it is okay, and not so scary, to be changing." Following group sessions, she slept more soundly. Ultimately, her purging and cutting behaviors ended completely.*

The Feldenkrais Method takes adults back to infancy, mobilizing developmental processes at a fundamental level. "Through manualized movement sequencing a process of organic learning is stimulated which enables a sort of post-maturation and leads to the formation and integration of new, more functionally appropriate responses. The progression and promotion of the kinesthetic sense is, as our first and basic ability to perceive, deeply connected with our self-identity" [36].

7.1.1.2 Feldenkrais Functional Integration© as part of mainstream BN practice

> *As an adjunct to psychotherapy, I engaged Lana in a hands-on Feldenkrais Functional Integration "lesson," described as such for its being a form of nervous system education. Having spent many months in residential treatment facilities, Lana, who had been sexually abused by her grandfather from ages 3 to 8, suffered from BN-restricting type with co-occurring bi-polar disorder type II, fibromyalgia, substance abuse, promiscuity, and self-mutilation. Though human touch is typically a delicate issue for victims of sexual abuse, through our secure 2-year therapeutic attachment and her trust in the healing process, she described my hands-on work as "a comfort, helping me to feel myself directly, and to feel myself in control." Through these lessons, she began to discern parallels between her undifferentiated expressions of emotional rage, and her body's undifferentiated and painful immobility during fibromyalgia flare-ups. As her body became increasingly flexible, differentiated, and ultimately re-integrated through her movement experiences she became more adept at differentiating and reintegrating her emotions as well, becoming calmer and increasingly regulated. Lana spoke of her Feldenkrais experience as "clearing out the cobwebs in my brain." At the end of one Feldenkrais session, in response to my lifting her leg off the treatment table in order to assess her degree of neuro-skeletal integration, Lana described feeling a sense of "overwhelming relief and gratitude" for the now seemingly apparent weightlessness in her leg, in contrast with her own self-perception. "This is the first time I can remember feeling good about living inside this body of mine"].*

Lana's sensation of physiological lightness was the result of her brain having uploaded novel sensory information through her newly reorganized nervous system. Embodied learning awakened Lana's sensory epiphany, followed by an increasingly integrated sense of self and identity. Though positive sensorimotor sensations might initially appear to be fleeting, the nervous system's brain and body 'own' these changes, with continued practice deepening the sustainability of learning and healing.

7.1.2 Sensorimotor interventions designed to address and heal trauma

A 2007 study revealed that trauma is significantly associated with the onset of ED, particularly BN and binge eating disorder. Traumatic experiences may include physical and emotional neglect (including food deprivation); physical, sexual, and emotional abuse and assault; teasing; and bullying [37]. The following are two additional forms of sensorimotor movement interventions shown to offer beneficial results for BN individuals who have experienced trauma.

7.1.2.1 Trauma-informed yoga

It is not unusual for ED individuals with restrictive eating disorders to attempt to control symptoms by using strenuous exercise to increase caloric expenditure. Trauma-informed yoga offers these individuals a safe avenue for the engagement in physical activity while providing an outlet for disease-associated symptoms [38]. Trauma-informed yoga reprograms the brain through activating novel movement, breathing, and action patterns and their psychological correlates. Facilitating sensorimotor processing and mitigating stress responses through combined top-down and bottom-up influences, yoga practice provides "a non-threatening means by which to unearth previously disavowed emotions stored in the 'emotional' limbic system, then cortically mediates traumatic pathways and thoughts through psychological appraisal methods" [38]. Teaching the use of breath facilitates close attention to present-moment awareness of self, bringing the nervous system from a dysregulated state to a unified, centered state by shifting the sympathetic nervous system to a balanced parasympathetic sense of calm and relaxation, while offering patients a sustainable relationship with the internal body. [39] By associating bodily states with emotional experiences, yoga gives rise to conscious feelings that occur through changes in the nervous system, fostering increased interoceptive awareness, thereby increasing emotional regulation in response to negative affect [22].

7.1.2.2 Eye Movement Desensitization and Reprocessing (EMDR)

Given the correlation between trauma and the onset of BN, Eye Movement Desensitization and Reprocessing (EMDR) offers an alternative interpersonal, experiential and body-centered therapy approach that treats the BN patient's co-occurring PTSD. Through EMDR, the patient processes and resolves sensations and emotions connected to traumatic memory stored in the limbic brain. The technique uses a unique procedure in which the therapist exposes the patient to rhythmic bilateral stimulation (BLS), using alternating bilateral visual (eye movement), auditory, or sensory stimulation [40], (e.g., tactile stimulation, such as the therapist's sequential touching of the patient's right knee and left knee). The technique relieves affective distress, reformulates negative beliefs and reduces physiological arousal. EMDR allows faster and more highly effective processing for trauma than does psychotherapy, as the neural substrate of rhythmic movement has more direct links to the limbic system than to language-based regions. Once disseminated (dissociated) fragments of traumatic memory have been reconnected, they become capable of integrating a new personal semantic memory network with new cognitive schemas, thus fulfilling the goal of EMDR treatment [41].

8. The neurobiology of mindful human attachment repairs impaired self-structure

"Energy and information can flow within the brain and between brains, profoundly shaping the flow of energy and information within and between people" [13]. The self-organization of the infant's developing brain occurs in the context of a relationship with another self, another brain" [42]. Allan Schore defines psychotherapy as "an attachment relationship that affects underlying neuronal structure and function" [43]. His developmental model places particular emphasis upon "the experience-dependent maturation of a system in the orbital prefrontal cortex that regulates psychophysiological state and organismic energy balance" [43]. "When the therapist's mind and embodied-self come together in relationship with those of the patient, implicit systems of the therapist interact with implicit systems of the patient, rendering psychotherapy the 'talking' cure. Talking to neurons alters neuronal networks and the functional sphere of influence of the prefrontal lobes" [16].

"By means of reverie and intuition, the sensitive empathic clinician's monitoring of unconscious process, rather than content, calls for right brain attention to matching the patient's implicit affective-arousal states, a process that lies at the core of the therapeutic relationship. Through the subconscious processing of information, the clinician uses an expansive attention mechanism that includes free association, while the left brain, more involved in the conscious processing of information, focuses on local detail" [43]. The resulting 'empathic resonance' is an embodied, sensed connection, typically experienced between therapist and patient as a dynamic, spirited, vibrant, and often loving mutual attachment, in which the patient's right brain hemisphere becomes altered in form and function in response to a mindful, energetic connection with the therapist's right brain hemisphere. Resonance exists 'outside our skin,' giving rise to a therapy relationship in which 'a mind is being changed by a mind'" [44] Deeply ensconced in psychophysiology, empathic resonance may be considered 'sharing a common brain,' with the intersubjective field between two individuals including far more than two minds, to include two bodies" [45].

According to Schore, "emotional healing takes place primarily in the circuitry of the right brain hemisphere, which is dominant for attachment, intense emotionality, and the knowledge of how to be in relationships' [46]. "Right brain to right brain emotional processes are central to emotional development, psychopathology, and psychotherapy. The functions of the emotional right brain foster the self-exploration process of psychotherapy, especially of unconscious affects that can be integrated into a more complex and implicit sense of self. Emotional communication between therapist and patient lies at the psychobiological core of the therapeutic alliance. Therapist affect facilitation is a powerful predictor of treatment success" [47]. Studies show that the more successful the treatment, the greater the neuroplastic change [48].

The brain's mirror neuron system is the foundational building block for empathy, a major component of healthy [resonant] psychotherapeutic attachment. Leading to a new theory of empathy that is bottom-up and top-down in nature, "mirror neurons reveal the fundamental integration within the brain of the perceptual and motor systems with limbic and somatic regulatory functions" [27]. It is through the therapist's empathy and genuine caring that patients come to feel listened to, heard, seen for who they are, and even loved, sometimes for the first time in their lives.

> *Thinking back, Tess revealed that after our first therapy session, she felt frightened, yet at the same time, compelled to continue treatment. "It was as though you could see right through me. It was terrifying for me to feel so totally transparent to you, with all of my defects. Yet at the same time it was thrilling for me that you actually saw goodness in me, strengths and even excellence in parts of my life, none of which I had ever before recognized. I was afraid that you would eventually see through to my inadequacies and feel repelled by me, rejecting me as your patient. As the weeks passed, I knew in my heart that this would be the only chance I'd ever have, to understand who I am and who I could become, why I am sick, and how to get better so that my life could become my own for the first time ever"].*

"It is through the relationship that deficits in internal working models of the self and the world are gradually repaired" [43].

8.1 The therapist's versatile and empathic use of self fosters patient self-reintegration

For BN individuals who failed to experience the benefits of healthy attachment during childhood, an effective therapeutic attachment offers a second real-time opportunity to feel the intrapersonal gratification that can be derived from a secure and trusting interpersonal attachment relationship with another human being. The healing therapeutic relationship becomes the prototype for healthful, quality relationships, both within, and beyond, the treatment dyad. "The highest human functions... including stress regulation, humor, empathy, compassion... are all right brain functions. An expanded capacity for right, not left, brain processing lies at the core of clinical expertise" [46]. The skillful and knowledgeable psychotherapist needs to maintain a mindful, pro-active and viable presence within each therapy moment, using himself or herself with intention, versatility, flexibility, courage, intuition and creativity [49]. Because ED represent changes within neural systems that mediate reward responses, decision-making, and social behaviors, effective treatment requires individualization based upon the specific constellation of symptoms presented, as well as their neurobiological underpinnings. As psycho-educators, practitioners need to keep patients informed about anticipated neurobiological changes in brain function related to impaired nutrition, such as fatigue, concentration and learning deficits, mood swings, insomnia, and impulsivity [2]. Patients also need to become aware of the positive changes in brain function that occur side-by-side with, and as result of, BN recovery.

The therapist's openness to his or her own bodily state is a crucial requirement for establishing interpersonal attunement with the patient [27]. "The therapist who is not intimidated, and who feels comfortable disclosing his or her own self-experience in appropriate, boundaried and clearly intentional ways, offers patients the opportunity and permission to bring forward more of their own seemingly intolerable experience. Therapist receptivity assures patients that they need not censor themselves, so that difficult emotions lose some of their threat" [44]. For purposes of role modeling in promoting the patient's learning and self-discovery, the clinician's self-revelation potentially fills gaps in the patient's emotional and self-development. Immediate, in-the-moment inquiry about the patient's counter-transferential reactions to the therapist's disclosure enhances the patient's sensing of self-experience and interpersonal trust building. "So, what's it like for you that I have chosen to share this information with you today?" "As an interactive regulator of the patient's psychological state" [47], the therapist's trust in, and acknowledgment of, the patient's strengths, resiliency, and potential to achieve recovery inspires and sustains the patient's belief in herself, fortifying her capacity to withstand the challenges of navigating the BN recovery process...as well as life without an ED.

Secure attachment relationships are based in mutual trust.

Emma shared, "You are the first person who has ever really listened to me, seeing beneath the surface to who I really am." Feeling stressed for having to leave town and therapy for several weeks, she texted me from afar about her disappointment in herself for having purged. "I hope I am not intruding on your time in reaching you like this," she wrote. "I genuinely care about you, and am glad to hear from you whenever and however it works best." I replied. "It is important for you to understand that the 'failure' you describe is not a failure at all, but a normal part of every stage of the recovery process. Knowing you as I do, I trust that you will continue to go from strength to strength, just as you've done your entire life, from early childhood onwards. And, if you are assessing the quality of your recovery,

> *please don't forget to consider the newfound clarity of your empowered voice in communicating with your husband, and his response, which has been respectful and loving in return. I look forward to one day soon when you will begin to recognize your own growing strengths and much deserved self-trust. She responded, "Thanks. You're right. I appreciate your thoughts."*

"Because empathy accounts for as much, and probably more, outcome variance than does the specific intervention, the quality of the therapy alliance is more important to treatment outcomes than the particular treatment method or theory embraced by the therapist" [48]. This becomes increasingly so, as patients internalize and own dyadic gains.

> *Trust-building secures therapeutic relationships outside the professional office.*

> *Tess had planned to observe a religious holiday that would have required a day's fasting. Prior to the holiday, between therapy sessions, it occurred to me that she might consider the alternative of reframing her commitment to observance this year by spending this day eating healthfully, instead. I phoned her to share my thoughts. "You think about me outside our sessions?! That's the best gift you could ever give me!" She was proud to report having been successful at fulfilling this unique challenge.*

The therapist's clearly defined boundaries and skilled navigation of complex transference and countertransference issues are essential in reinforcing the effective use of self in what, in some instances, becomes a process similar to re-parenting. In reinforcing a loving, secure, healthy, and trusted attachment, the therapist re-visits, refreshes, and re-inspires the patient's healthfully continuing self-development.

9. Trauma resolution occurs through neurobiological reintegration of the distributed nervous system

Independent of its etiology, any traumatic assault on, or insult to, the brain impairs brain integration. A recent study found that "the vast majority of women and men with AN and BN reported a history of interpersonal trauma, with approximately one-third of BN women meeting criteria for lifetime PTSD [50]. Another study reported that sexual abuse occurs in 30–65% of women with ED, and that women with BN and substance dependence disorder had the highest frequency and most severe history of sexual abuse [51]. High stress levels leading to an overactive amygdala and hippocampus suppress the activities of the prefrontal cortex...the thinking brain, that helps to regulate the emotional brain.

The psychosomatic expressions of trauma experiences are held as bodily sensations, which become embedded in a broad variety of psychopathological and intersubjective phenomena [52]. Unprocessed traumatic memories stored in the mid-brain region become recycled when triggered, creating undischarged energy in the nervous system. Because traumatic memories are encoded subcortically, the process of healing trauma requires gaining leverage within the structural coding of the brain. Psychotherapeutic "'interpretation'" has been shown to have limited effectiveness with pathologies arising from the verbal phase related to explicit memories, and no effect on the pre-verbal phase implicit memories" [52]. Trauma speaks through the body. Trauma has been described as a "disorder of arousal." Its resolution lies in creating a psychophysiological state associated with decreased adrenergic activity, decreased muscular neuromuscular arousal, and cognitive quieting [53].

Rapid Resolution Therapy (RRT), illustrated in the examples in Section 9.1, is a body-based talk therapy technique shown to alleviate negative effects of trauma and PTSD without requiring the patient to recollect painful memories. Within the context of a trusted relationship, the technique connects problems to solutions through the human nervous system by consolidating memories of past and present human strengths and resourcefulness [54]. “Trauma resides in the limbic system (responsible for emotional systems and defensive responses) and in the perceptual world within a neural network that has sufficient functional boundary thresholds to largely ‘dis-integrate’ it from the rest of the nervous system. When negative feelings become dissociated or ‘split off’ [as they do with the bulimic pseudo-self], the potential exists to reintegrate them through the patient’s connection with a better state, her best self, by sensing and owning her resourceful self through solution-discovery, or rediscovery, both past and present” [33]. Trauma resolution “accesses neuroplasticity, through which neural networks that become lit-up at the same time as the neural network associated with the problem, result in the problem’s loss of definition. This dynamic allows for a free flow of communication with the rest of the nervous system, as the brain re-interprets new combinations of neural connections to create meaning” [54]. Because the effects of past trauma are revealed in the present, they become accessible, and thereby, available for remediation.

9.1 Sensing, recall, and consolidation of resourcefulness memories heal trauma

Trauma occupies the right side of the brain where it creates a hyperactive cortisol network; the processing of trauma needs to occur within the left side of the brain, where some form of resolution can be reached. The healing process becomes reinforced through connections to real-life experience, as the therapist guides the patient to access her already existing internal resourcefulness.

> *Having grown up in a dysfunctional, chaotic family environment during which her father spent years in prison, Lillian is a highly functioning divorced woman struggling with BN, depression, anxiety, and alcohol addiction. Her impaired self-perception, self-regulation, and distrust in her judgment and decision-making have kept her resentfully tied to a long-term, disorganized relationship with a boyfriend upon whom she relies to provide compensatory external controls. Though considering herself to be “helpless and hopeless,” this day she spoke of her excellent performance in her new job, the gratifying relationships she’d established there, and her improved relationship with her adolescent son. “When you are feeling good about such experiences, have you ever sensed where inside your body you notice sensations of pleasure or gratification?” I asked. She had not noticed. I invited her to probe her sensory recall, calling up past fulfilling experiences where she might have sensed an internal body-felt ‘lightness of being.’ She could not. Upon parting, she randomly commented that the Botanic Garden in which we had walked and talked that day had offered a delightful and uplifting experience. Capturing that opportunity, I replied, “Try to observe where in your body you might be sensing your positive feelings now, right at this moment.” Lillian pointed to her heart. “Perhaps the next time you notice yourself feeling inadequate, out of control or fearful, you might want to try to bring up your body’s sensory memory of your feelings of contentment right now, in this beautiful place. You might just come to discover that the same body that has long been your worst enemy could possibly become your greatest ally”.*

Tapping into old ‘feel good’ moments facilitates positivity in the experience of now.

“Eating disorders, which are dysfunctions of multisensory body integration, are the outcome of primary disturbances in the way the body is “experienced” and "remembered" [55]. Memory consolidation puts the experience of body phenomena into the thinking brain, securing it there through the creation and re-creation of healthy neurobiological circuitry and neuronal connections between mind, brain, and body.

> *A 6-year-old Honduran child, whose mother had brought him to the U.S. seeking asylum, underwent sustained trauma during his one-month detention in a cage at the country's border, separated from his mother. Having seen a film clip of their reunion on television, Tess watched the agonized child convulsing and crying in anguish and recrimination. "You gave me away. You don't love me. You are not my mom anymore, and I don't want to be your son. I want to go back to the jail." Tess, having been abused and neglected by her own mother, instantaneously succumbed to re-experiencing her own traumatic childhood feelings of rejection. She purged immediately after viewing the program and awoke the following morning with an aching body, and a pain that "took up all the space in my stomach." In an emergency therapy session that morning, Tess sat on my couch with bent knees tightly drawn up to her chin, arms tightly encircling her legs, her body language expressing a somatic narrative that portrayed fear and the need for self-protection. She described her previous night's experience, "where my dissociated bulimic self harangued me about how repulsive, despicable and worthless I am. I became painfully aware that all of my progress in treatment had gone up in smoke, becoming 'unreal' to me, as though it never happened." During our treatment session, Tess became aware of how her mother currently and consistently continues to fuel her shame and psychic pain, into the present. She also became able to recognize her own co-dependent fear and reluctance to erect a viable emotional boundary between them. Having become fully present in the here and now within our secure attachment, our solution-based dialogue during that session countered her right-brain activation by creating a coherent, left-brain narrative, consolidating and reintegrating more recent body-felt remembrances of her healthy Self. Within two hours time, her face and body had visibly relaxed to a state of calm as she shifted out of the past into the fulfillment and gratification of her present life. Tess left that session with a smile on her face, expressing an overwhelming sense of relief and gratitude.*

Tess's successful resolution of this traumatic incident held out the promise of change within her nervous system reflecting a greater and more spontaneous capacity to access her internal resiliency in the face of future resurgences of traumatic memory. The process of trauma resolution in working with BN patients is no different from healing trauma in any other context, with the exception that in light of the integrative nature of an ED, attention to trauma resolution needs to become part of a greater fabric of pathology, all aspects of which demand resolution and healing if ED recovery is to be complete and sustainable.

10. Conclusion

Characterized by biochemical, neuromuscular, and sensory imbalances, BN fosters internal chaos and system rigidity, disrupting the integrity of the patient's core self. Clinicians and patients alike need to understand and anticipate that BN treatment and recovery processes are never linear. Tess describes her treatment as being "highly successful…my eating lifestyle, coping abilities, relationships, life quality, and over-all sense of well-being have all significantly improved…yet my BN is still and always lurking within arm's reach, capable of stopping me in my tracks when I am least expecting it." Integrative disorders demand integrative treatment approaches.

The capacity for self-correction is built into the nervous system through the brain's ability to integrate sensing, perception, and motor activity. Effective treatment needs to support changes at the brain level, with attention paid to mental, somatic, and relational issues. The creation of neural firing patterns that awaken the brain enables newly established synaptic connections, promoting self-awareness of one's internal world, which modulates and modifies it [27], promoting self-integration.

According to Allan Schore, a significant paradigm shift in psychotherapy is occurring, marked by clinical modes now moving from left brain to right brain, from the mind to the body, and from the central to the autonomic nervous system [52]. "After three decades of cognitive approaches, motivational and emotional processes have roared back into the limelight...cognitive interventions have been proven short-lived in their efficacy, and limited in the problems to which they can be applied" [47]. The right hemisphere is dominant in the change process of psychotherapy. Body-based right brain affect, including specifically unconscious affect, is best accessed through updated, adjunctive psychotherapeutic interventions [47]. Psychobiological attachment-based empathic resonance between the patient and therapist, and the use of adjunctive top-down and bottom-up neurophysiological interventions in appropriate situations and with clarity of intention, address the neurobiological roots of disease, beyond symptoms, in fostering mind, brain, and body connections that promote integration of the structure of the self.

Though we live in an era of psychotherapy research and practice where specific modes of psychotherapeutic treatment have been recognized as targeting specific sites of brain functioning [56], mainstream clinical eating disorder treatment continues to focus on symptom reduction alone, neglecting the neurological origins and underpinnings of these disorders. Clinicians need to become better prepared to resolve these lethal disorders at their source by accessing the brain and distributed nervous system, fostering the sustainability of ameliorative change. In so doing, they stand on the precipice of a new age of treatment, moving patients, the field, and eating disorder research, forward.

Acknowledgements

Heartfelt thanks and gratitude go to my dear friend and fellow writer, Lyn Haber, whose brilliant edits and much-appreciated tenacity were so supportive and uplifting to me throughout this project.

Many thanks go to 'Tess,' for having provided astute insights and contributions as I put this chapter together. As a soon-to-be psychotherapist herself, and a joy and pleasure to have worked with in treatment, she has my love, respect, and gratitude.

Abbreviations

AN	anorexia nervosa
BN	bulimia nervosa
ED	eating disorders
CBT	cognitive-behavioral therapy
EMDR	eye movement desensitization and reprocessing
RRT	rapid resolution therapy
ATM	awareness through movement
FI	functional integration
PTSD	post-traumatic stress disorder
BLS	bilateral stimulation

Author details

Abigail H. Natenshon
Eating Disorder Specialists of Illinois, Highland Park, Illinois, USA

*Address all correspondence to: abigailnatenshon@gmail.com

References

[1] Russell G. Bulimia Nervosa: An ominous variant of anorexia nervosa. Psychological Medicine. 1979;**9**(3):429-424

[2] Kaye WH, Fudge JL, Paulus M. New insights into symptoms and neurocircuit function of anorexia nervosa. Nature Reviews Neuroscience. 2009;**10**(8): 573-584. DOI: 10.1038/nrn2682

[3] Russell R. Movement and the development of sense of self. In: Proceedings from the International Conference on the Feldenkrais Method; August 2004; Seattle, Washington.

[4] Kaye W. Neurobiology of anorexia and bulimia nervosa purdue ingestive behavior research center symposium influences on eating and body weight over the lifespan: Children and adolescents. Physiology & Behavior. 2008;**94**(1):121-135. DOI: 10.1016/j.physbeh.2007.11.037

[5] Mickalide AD, Anderson AE. Subgroups of anorexia nervosa and bulimia: Validity and utility. Journal of Psychiatric Research. 1985;**19**(2-2):121-128

[6] Whiteman H. Why are women more vulnerable to eating disorders? Brain study sheds light. Medical News Today. 2016

[7] Moseman S. Understanding Neurobiology and Eating Disorders. Tulsa, Oklahoma: Laureate Eating Disorders Program; 2014. http://www.eatingdisorderhope.com/treatment-for-eating-disorders/types-of-treatments/neurobiology-can-play-key-role-in-treating-eating-disorders

[8] Via E, Zalesky A, Sanchez I, Forcano L, Harrison BJ, Pujol J, et al. Disruption of brain white matter microstructure in women with anorexia nervosa. Journal of Psychiatry & Neuroscience. 2014;**39**(6):367-375. DOI: 10.1503/jpn.130135

[9] University of Illinois at Chicago. Abnormalities found in 'Insight' Areas of the Brain in Anorexia. ScienceDaily. 2016. www.sciencedaily.com/releases/2016/07/160719123857.htm

[10] Frank G. Eating disorders impact brain function, new brain research suggests. Science News. University of Colorado Denver; 2011. https://www.sciencedaily.com/releases/2011/07/110711144944.htm

[11] Reindl SM. Sensing the Self: Women's Recovery from Bulimia. Cambridge, MA: Harvard University Press; 2001

[12] Bruch H. Eating Disorders. Obesity, Anorexia Nervosa and the Person Within. New York: Basic Books, Inc., Publishers; 1973

[13] National Institute for the Clinical Application of Behavioral Medicine NICABM. Master Strategies in the Treatment of Trauma: The Latest Interventions can Reduce Symptoms and Speed Healing [Internet]. 2018. Available from: https://www.nicabm.com/tag/treating-trauma-master-series/ [Accessed:2018-11-07]

[14] Siegel DJ. How to Understand your Mind [Internet]. Leadership Online Training Program; 2017

[15] Siegel DJ. Mindsight: The New Science of Personal Transformation. New York: Bantam/Random House; 2010

[16] Doidge N. The Brain that Changes Itself: Stories of Personal Triumph from the Frontiers of Brain Science. New York: Viking; 2007

[17] Feldenkrais M. Awareness through Movement: Health Exercises for Personal Growth. New York: Harper and Row; 1972

[18] Doidge N. The Brain's Way of Healing: Remarkable Recoveries and Discoveries from the Frontiers of Neuroplasticity. New York: Viking; 2015

[19] Cheever OL, Cohen LJ, Leskowitz E. In: Micozzi MS, editor. The Feldenkrais Method; Complementary and Alternative Medicine in Rehabilitation. USA: Elsevier Science; 2003. pp. 39-50

[20] Feldenkrais M. Embodied Wisdom: The Collected Papers of Moshe Feldenkrais. Beringer ed. Berkeley, CA: Somatic Awareness and North Atlantic Books; 2010

[21] Price CJ, Hooven C. Interoceptive awareness skills for emotion regulation: Theory and approach of mindful awareness in body-oriented therapy (MABT). Frontiers in Psychology. 2018;**9**:798. DOI: 10.3389/fpsyg.2018.00798

[22] Fustos J, Gramann K, Herbert BM, Pollatos O. On the embodiment of emotion regulation: Interoceptive awareness facilitates reappraisal. Social Cognitive and Affective Neuroscience. 2013;**8**(8):911-917. DOI: 10.1093/scan/nss089

[23] Ionta S, Gassert R, Blanke O. Multi-sensory and sensorimotor foundation of bodily self-consciousness—An interdisciplinary approach. Frontiers in Psychology. 2011;2:383. DOI: 10.3389/fpsyg.so11.00383

[24] de Vos AJ, Lamarre A, Radstaak M, Bijkirk CA, Bohlmeijer E, Westerhof GJ. Identifying fundamental criteria for eating disorder recovery: A systematic review and qualitative meta-analysis. Journal of Eating Disorders. 2017;**5**(1): 1-14. DOI: 10.1186-s40337-017-0164-0

[25] Hill L, Knatz Peck S, Wierenga CE, Kaye WH. Applying neurobiology to the treatment of adults with anorexia nervosa. Journal of Eating Disorders. 2016;**4**(31):1-14. DOI: 10.1186/s40337-016-0119-x

[26] Riva G. the neuroscience of body memory: From the self through the space to the others. Cortex. 2017;**104**:241-260. DOI: 10.1016/J.Cortx.2017.07.013

[27] Siegel DJ. An interpersonal neurobiology approach to psychotherapy; awareness, mirror neurons, and neural plasticity in the development of well-being. Psychiatric Annals. 2006;**36**(4):248-256

[28] Sze JA, Gyurak A, Yuan JW, Levenson RW. Coherence between emotional experience and physiology: Does body awareness training have an impact? Emotion. 2010;**10**(6):803-814

[29] OpenPSYC. Openpsyc.blogspot.com/2014/06booem

[30] Taylor AG, Goehler LE, Galper DI, Innes KE, Bourguignon C. Top-down and bottom-up mechanisms in mind-body medicine: Development of an integrative framework for psychophysiological research. Explore. 2010;**6**(1):29. DOI: 10.1016/j.explore.2011.12.005

[31] Fuglset TM, Landro NI, Reas DL, Ro O. Functional brain alterations in anorexia nervosa: A scoping review. Journal of Eating Disorders. 2016;**4**(32):1-13. DOI: 10.1186/s40337-016-0118-y

[32] Janowiak-Siuda K, Rymarczyk K, Grabowska A. How we empathize with others: A neurobiological perspective. Medical Science Monitor. 2011;**17**(1):RA18-RA24. DOI: 10.12659/msm.881324

[33] Connelly J. The Institute for Rapid Resolution Therapy. https://www.floridacenterforrecovery.com/addiction-glossary/rapid-resolution-therapy

[34] Ogden P, Pain C, Fisher J. A sensorimotor approach to the

treatment of trauma and dissociation. Psychiatric Clinics of North America. 2006;**29**(1):263-279, xi-xii. DOI: 10.1016/j.psc.2005.10.012

[35] Eshkebari E, Rieger E, Longo M, Haggard P, Treasure J. Persistent body image disturbance following recovery from eating disorders. The International Journal of Eating Disorders. 2014;**47**:400-409

[36] Laumer U, Bauer M, Fichter M, Milz H. Therapeutic effects of the feldenkrais method (awareness through movement) in eating disorders. IFF Academy: Feldenkrais Research Journal. 2004;**1**:2

[37] Brewerton TD. Eating disorders, trauma, and comorbidity: Focus on PTSD. Journal of Treatment and Prevention. 2007;**15**(4):285-304 www.nationaleatingdisorders.org/blog/eating-disorders-trauma-ptsd-recovery

[38] Hall A, Ofei-Tenkorang NA, Machn JT, Gordon CM. Use of yoga in outpatient eating disorder treatment: A pilot study. Journal of Eating Disorders. 2016;**4**(38):1-8. DOI: 10.1186/s40337-016-0130-2

[39] Kinser P, Goehler L, Taylor AG. How might yoga heal depression? A neurological perspective. Explore. 2012;**8**(2):118. DOI: 10.1016/j.explore.2011.12.005

[40] Korn D, Leeds AM. Preliminary evidence of efficacy of EMDR resource development and installation in the stabilization phase of treatment of complex posttraumatic stress disorder. Journal of Clinical Psychology. 2002;**58**(12):1465-1487

[41] Coubard OA. Eye movement desensitization and reprocessing (EMDR) reexamined as cognitive and emotional neuroentertainment. Frontiers in Human Neuroscience. 2015;**8**:1035. DOI: 10.3398/fnhum.2014.01035

[42] Mahler MS, Pine F, Bergman A. The Psychological Birth of the Human Infant: Symbiosis and Individuation. New York: Basic Books; 1931

[43] Schore AN. The experience-dependent maturation of a regulatory system in the orbital prefrontal cortex and the origin of developmental psychopathology. Development and Psychopathology. 1996;**8**:59-87

[44] Schore JR, Schore AN. Modern attachment theory: The central role of affect regulation in development and treatment. Clinical Social Work Journal. 2008;**36**(1):9-20. DOI: 10.1007/s10615-007-0111-7

[45] Schore AN. Early organization of the non-linear right brian and development of the predisposition to psychiatric disorders. Development and Psychopathology. 1996;**8**(1):59-87

[46] Halasz G. In conversation with allan schore. Australian Psychiatry. 2011;**19**(1):30-36. DOI: 10.3109/10398562.2010.530757

[47] Schore AN. Right brain affect regulation: An essential mechanism of development, trauma, dissociation, and psychotherapy. In: Fosha D, Siegel DJ, Solomon M, editors. Papers by YellowBrick Leadership. The Healing Power of Emotion: Affective Neuroscience, Development, and Clinical Practice. New York City: WW Norton; 2009

[48] Germer CK, Siegel RD, Fulton PR. Mindfulness and Psychotherapy. Guilford Press; 2005

[49] Natenshon A. Eating disorders: A treatment apart. In: Jauregui-Lobera, editor. Eating Disorders: A Paradigm of the Biopsychosocial Model of Illness. Intech; 2017. pp. 165-187

[50] Mitchell KS, Mazzeo SE, Schlesinger MR, Brewerton TD,

Smith BN. Comorbidity of partial and subthreshold PTSD among men and women with eating disorders in the National Comorbidity Survey-Replication Study. The International Journal of Eating Disorders. 2012;**45**(3):307-315. DOI: 10.1002/eat.20965

[51] Deep AL, Lilenfeld LR, Plotnicov KH, Pollice C, Kaye WH. Sexual abuse in eating disorder subtypes and control women: The role of comorbid substance dependence in bulimia nervosa. The International Journal of Eating Disorders. 1999;**25**:1-10

[52] Ogden P, Pain C, Minton K, Fisher J. In: Schore AN, editor. Including the Body in Mainstream Psychotherapy for Traumatized Individuals. Vol. 25(4). Psychologist-Psychoanalyst. 2005. Retrieved from: http://www.sensorimotorpsychotherapy.org/article%20APA.html

[53] Everly GS Jr, Benson H. Disorders of arousal and the relaxation response: Speculations on the nature and treatment of stress-related diseases. International Journal of Psychosomatics. 1989;**36**(1-4):15-21

[54] Quintal JS. Trauma resolution treatment...and more; rhizomatics and the processes of change. In: Proceedings of the SelahFreedom: Bringing Light into the Darkness of Sex Trafficking. Conference; 8-9 November 2018; Winnetka, Illinois. p. 4

[55] Riva G, Gaudio S. Locked to the wrong body: Eating disorders are the outcome of a primary disturbance in multisensory body integration. Consciousness and Cognition. 2018;**59**:57-59

[56] Gabbard GO. A neurobiologically informed perspective on psychotherapy. The British Journal of Psychiatry. 2000;**1777**:117-122. www.ncbi.nlm.nih.gov/pubmed/11026950

Chapter 10

Severe and Enduring Eating Disorders: Concepts and Management

Paul Robinson

Abstract

The concept of severe and enduring mental illness was introduced in 1999 in order to direct resources to patients suffering from long-term serious disorders, and was suggested for eating disorders in 2009. However, the term is still restricted to patients with long-term psychosis. In this chapter, the concept of severe and enduring eating disorder (SEED) is described and its relevance to anorexia nervosa (AN) and bulimia nervosa (BN) is explored. The recovery curve for anorexia nervosa seems to follow an exponential pattern with an asymptote that approaches but does not meet the horizontal, suggesting that recovery is always possible. Symptoms of AN but not BN seem to worsen after 3 years of illness, perhaps a significant threshold. Symptoms of severe and enduring AN (SEED-AN) are debilitating and longstanding as well as potentially fatal. Symptoms of severe and enduring BN (SEED-BN) are also debilitating, especially in social adjustment. In both conditions, family difficulties are prominent. A clinical approach to SEED is described based on improving quality of life, the recovery approach, (rather than cure) for sufferers and their families is described, although full symptomatic recovery can occur at any stage and clinicians should be alert to the possibility in all patients.

Keywords: anorexia nervosa, bulimia, chronic, severe and enduring, recovery model

1. Introduction

The idea of severe and enduring mental illness (SEMI) extends back to 1999 when the UK Department of Health published the National Service Framework [1]. In it, SEMI was defined as follows:

> *"People with recurrent or severe and enduring mental illness, for example schizophrenia, bipolar affective disorder or organic mental disorder, severe anxiety disorders or severe eating disorders, have complex needs which may require the continuing care of specialist mental health services working effectively with other agencies."*

Clearly it was intended, rightly, to include non-psychotic disorders such as eating disorders and obsessive-compulsive disorder. Since that time policy has changed, perhaps because of increasing demands on community psychiatric services due to bed closures and funding restrictions and the most recent definition is very restrictive. In 2018, the National Institute for Clinical and Care Excellence (NICE) [2] released the draft scope for SEMI and stated: "the groups that will be covered are *Adults (aged 18 years and older) with complex psychosis*". Ruggeri et al. [3] provided two sets of criteria that reflect this tension: 1. Diagnosis of psychosis, 2. Duration of service contact ≥2 years, 3. GAF (Global Assessment of Functioning) score, <50 and a second model only including the latter two criteria, hence including non-psychotic disorders (including eating disorders).

In this context in which access to services could be restricted by psychiatric teams on the basis that the patient did not have a severe and enduring mental illness, the author wrote a book entitled Severe and Enduring Eating Disorders [4] partly in an attempt to draw attention to the ongoing major problems experienced by people with long term eating disorders. In this chapter we will examine the SEMI concept as applied to eating disorders, review the symptoms experienced by SEED patients and look at the differences between different eating disorders, which have lasted for many years. In the last section, recommendations for management of SEED will be made.

2. Definitions and concepts

Eating disorders have been fully described in the DSM 5 [5] and these definitions will not be considered here. However, the questions of duration and severity do give rise to controversy and although the term Severe and Enduring" has been applied to eating disorders [4, 6], the precise length of history and severity required are still undecided.

2.1 Length of illness

This can be approached in a number of ways. One is to ask the question: At what point do eating disorders become significantly harder to treat? This is an important question, because if we knew the answer, we could make all possible efforts to begin treatment before that point. Unfortunately there is rather little evidence to guide us, although it has been suggested [7] that after 3 years of illness, anorexia nervosa may become more intractable. This is based on a randomised controlled study of anorexia nervosa [8] in which patients with a length of history of restricting anorexia nervosa of <3 years did significantly better in family therapy than patients with a longer history. Another approach is to look at the proportion of patients who still fulfil criteria for the disorder at different times after onset. In **Table 1**, a number of studies in which this proportion is reported are displayed. In each study, the proportion of patients with a "poor outcome" is noted in the 5th column. The proportion includes all deaths, as well as patients with a poor outcome due to reasons other than the eating disorder, so the measure is somewhat flawed. However, the proportion after 9–24 years (average 13.4 years) ranges from 12 to 59%, average 27.9%. This tells us that the proportion of patients initially diagnosed as having anorexia nervosa and who go on to do badly is high, and we can expect around a quarter of patients to follow this course. A more conservative estimate is shown in the 3rd column, namely the proportion of patients still fulfilling diagnostic criteria for anorexia nervosa. The range is from 3 to 37% with an average of 14.4%. The highest estimate in that column, 37% [13] is from a national service which accepted referrals from all over the UK. Hence the severity of disease in patients admitted is likely to be higher and length of illness proportionately longer.

Condition studied	Length of follow-up (years)	Proportion % fulfilling disease criteria	Notes	Poor outcome (ED and other reasons)	Reference
Anorexia nervosa	24	Diagnoses not recorded	Mortality 12.8%	29%	Theander et al. [9]
Anorexia nervosa	9	17	Mortality 11%	59%	Deter et al. [10]
Anorexia nervosa	12	19	Mortality 7.7%, BN 9.5%	39.6%	Fichter et al. [11]
Anorexia nervosa	10	3	Adolescents, no deaths, 5% BN, 23% personality disorder		Herpertz-Dahlmann et al. [12]
Anorexia nervosa	20	37	15% BN, 15% died	36.6%	Ratnasuriya et al. [13]
Anorexia nervosa	15	13	No deaths, 30% binge eating		Strober et al. [14]
Anorexia nervosa	10	6	Community screening, mean age onset 14	27%	Wentz et al. [15]
Anorexia nervosa	18	6	Same cohort as above	12%	Wentz et al. [16]
Average	13.4	14.4		27.9%	

Table 1.
Follow-up studies of anorexia nervosa.

Without that centre the average proportion fulfilling criteria at average 14 years is 9.14% which may be a more representative figure.

2.1.1 The asymptotic pattern of outcome

Four of the above studies [9–11, 16] provided data on outcome of anorexia nervosa at several time points which allows us to draw a survival curve (**Figure 1**).

This shows that as time goes on, the number of cases reduces and almost, but not quite, reaches the horizontal, that is the curve seems to represent an asymptote. It should be noted that at no time does the curve ever stop falling, although the gradient does flatten, showing that anorexia nervosa can always recover, at any stage. The graph suggests that significant flattening seems to occur between 5 and 10 years, and in that period after diagnosis recovery does become less likely. **Figure 1** also shows the exponential curve that was derived from the data points shown and this also suggests an asymptotic pattern.

2.1.2 Symptoms may increase in severity after 3 years

The proposal by Treasure and Russell [7] that a history of more than 3 years might be accompanied by a decreased responsiveness to treatment was further examined in a study by Gardini [17]. In this audit of routine questionnaires, results in patients with anorexia nervosa with under 3 years history were compared with a group of patients with a history of 3–10 years and a further group with over 10 years duration. A comparable study was performed for patients with a diagnosis of bulimia nervosa and the same durations of illness.

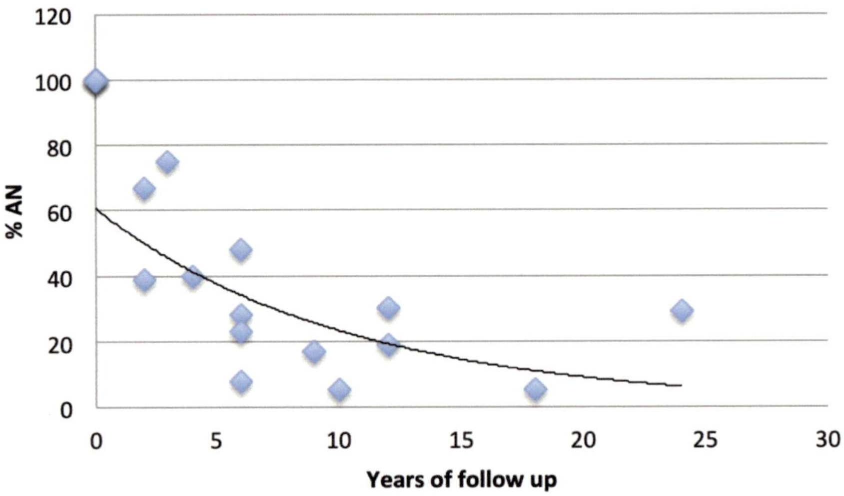

Figure 1.
Percentage of participants who fulfilled diagnostic criteria at each assessment from four follow-up studies of anorexia nervosa. The curve is exponential, derived from these data points.

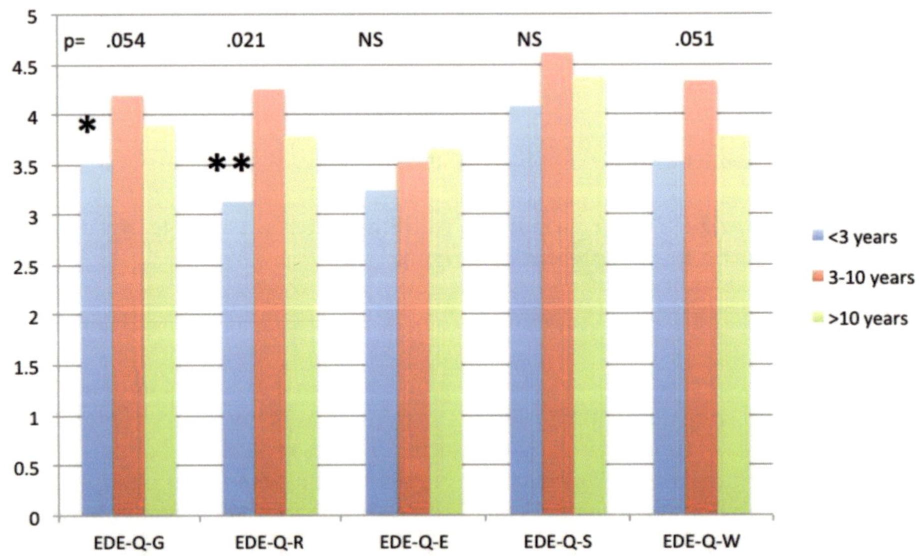

Figure 2.
*EDE-Q scores in three groups of patients with anorexia nervosa (total n = 87) with length of history of <3 years, 3–10 years and >10 years. The p values derive from a Manova comparing the three length of history groups. *≤3 years group vs. 3–10 year group p = 0.048, **≤3 years group vs. 3–10 year group p = 0.017 (post-hoc tests). EDE-Q-G: global score, EDE-Q-R: restraint, EDE-Q-E: eating concern, EDE-Q-S: shape concern, EDE-Q-W: weight concern.*

The results were intriguing. For anorexia nervosa (but not for bulimia nervosa), time had a significant impact on EDE-Q restraint and a borderline significant impact of EDE-Q weight concern and EDE-Q global score. The scores increased between <3 and 3–10 years and then declined after 10 years. The results are summarised in **Figure 2**.

This study provides some evidence for the 3 year threshold proposed by Treasure and Russell [7]. Some eating disorder symptoms significantly increase after 3 years illness and this could relate to increasing difficulty in helping patients achieve remission. The increased restraint score could reflect increased resistance to the parents encouraging the patient to consume a weight gaining diet, an essential element in family based therapy.

3. Clinical features of SEED

In this section, SEED-AN symptoms [18] will be compared with SEED-BN (unpublished data).

3.1 Physical

In SEED-AN, many participants complained of physical problems, but also denied their seriousness:

> *"The worst thing is going to be as I am moving in my latter years being osteoporotic but you know what, there are some fantastic tablets today."*

> *"Osteoporosis was diagnosed but I think it's controllable ... with Calcium and the right diet, and I think it's not acute."*

In SEED-BN most participants either did not complain of any physical problem, or felt they were manageable.

3.2 Psychological

In SEED-AN, most participants were depressed, and self esteem was often extremely low:

> *"I felt like I was a horrible, disgusting, person ... I felt like really ugly and disgusting and dirty and therefore to dress myself in things that made me look pretty would be like, it would be wrong somehow."*

In SEED-BN depression and mood instability were the rule.

> *"Sometimes I'm just bubbly and happy and in a fun mood and other days I just want to be on my own."*

> *"I think a lot of it is dealing with your depression."*

3.3 Social

In SEED-AN, social disruption, lack of intimate relationships and social isolation were common.

> *"I felt I just totally failed and dropped out of life. I was too scared to join up the squash club, I was too scared to socialise with people, I lost all my confidence with job interviews."*

In SEED-BN most participants were not in relationships and were living alone.

> *"I've got some friends that I have online but I haven't actually met them. Because I feel I can totally fake...see it kind of doesn't matter what I say because I haven't met them. Do you know what I mean? Because it doesn't matter if they disappear, they're not actually real friends."*

3.4 Family

In SEED-AN, the patient sometimes ended up as their parents' carer.

> *"I was sort of left; a lot of the family got married and moved away from home."*

In other cases, difficult relationships improved over time.

> *"In the last 2 years the relationship with my family has got better. I now have contact with my sister. We often chat on the phone. I don't really see my brothers or hear from them, I often ask my parents about them, they ask about me."*

In SEED-BN, family difficulties were frequent. Some felt their families did not take the eating disorder seriously. One patient after she had confessed her bulimia to her mother, reported that her mother said "*yeah I used to do it. It's so stupid. You kind of don't wanna do that ... ,*" which she did not find helpful. Other patients reported that their families were weight obsessed. When one participant had regained a size 12, a member of her extended family exclaimed "*Oh my God what have they been feeding you? You're enormous*!"

3.5 Financial

For SEED-AN, patients were often poor, living on benefits without paid work. They also described clinical frugality, in which they had extreme difficulty spending money on themselves:

> *"I find it very difficult spending money. If you walked into my flat, I've got nothing particular there ... just very-very bare. My shoes, I wear them until they begin to fall into pieces."*

For SEED-BN, the illness was often very costly because of the large quantity of food consumed. One patient interviewed was seeing a debt counsellor to manage loans from 5 different lenders: "*I don't have any savings, and I don't buy anything nice for myself, I just survive.*"

3.6 Occupational

SEED-AN: These patients often reported being out of work and surviving on benefits. "*I completed 1 year of that (teaching) course and then I had to go into hospital so that came to an end. ... I seemed to lose interest in work and it seemed more important that I planned my meals and my walks.*"

SEED-BN: These individuals were often in work, and some valued the structure of work to help manage their eating disorder: "*I feel that going to work in the morning 'wipes the slate clean' if I have binged and vomited the night before.*" Others found that the eating disorder had an adverse effect on work: "*Last summer I had to take a number of months off work due to my eating disorder and depression, and I still struggle to fulfill all my commitments when my mood is low.*"

4. Management

Outcome research in the area of management of SEED is sparse. There are several examples of publications in which clinicians have expressed their opinion in this area [14, 19, 20]. One question that constantly appears in the area of management is what general approach to use. As already discussed full recovery from an eating disorder is always possible although less likely as the years pass. The patient (and the clinician and family) are thus confronted with the question each time therapy is contemplated: Should I go for a full recovery or for the best quality-of-life given that I have a long-term disorder.

From the point of view of the clinician, there may be a moral dilemma. Funding for services may depend on inpatient units being full. This applies to both the public and private health sectors. There may therefore be perverse incentives to admit the SEED patient for a prolonged hospital stay in pursuit of weight gain. Most professionals in charge of an inpatient eating disorders service will be aware of these pressures, and how they sometimes conflict with patient care. Hospital admission is essential in the case of a patient who presents life threatening physical illness. However the likelihood of long-term recovery after prolonged admission in someone with a long illness is probably small and one is left with a suspicion that some SEED patients may be admitted for long periods without much benefit.

4.1 Cure or care?

It seems to the author evident that all patients with SEED to be offered treatment and that fully alleviating disorder. However not all patients benefit from this approach especially if it is provided against the patient's consent and in such cases a harm minimization or recovery approach focused on improving quality of life maybe more humane and helpful.

4.2 The recovery approach

This approach [21] that originated amongst service users in the United States posits that improved mental and physical health can be achieved even though the illness at the root of a person's difficulties cannot be cured. Thus a person with schizophrenia who hears voices, believes he is being bugged and has interpersonal difficulties can still be helped to deal with the symptoms through individual family and social interventions even though medication has had limited impact.

Can a similar approach applied to eating disorders? Here we will go through the different realms indicated by see patients as problematic and identify ways to approach them.

4.3 Medication

The role of medication in the eating disorders is limited and the main group who appear to benefit are those with bulimia nervosa. Antidepressants such as high-dose fluoxetine can be tried with patients who have had at least one evidence-based psychological treatment for bulimia nervosa [22]. Of other drugs olanzapine has been tried in anorexia nervosa [23] and although the evidence is currently weak, some eating disorder specialists believe that the drug reduces anxiety and may have an impact in improving weight gain. Adequate randomised trials are awaited.

4.4 Psychological therapy

Patients with anorexia nervosa and bulimia nervosa are in both quantitative and qualitative studies are found to suffer from depression and anxiety. These difficulties often correlate with the severity of the eating disorder symptoms such as lower weight or frequent bingeing and purging and treatments to reduce those are clearly the preferred approach. However patients with SEED have often received one or more courses of psychotherapy and perhaps one or more inpatient or day patient episodes. In anorexia nervosa there is little evidence that any therapy is better than any other although in bulimia nervosa CBT [24] and some other approaches have been found helpful. In a trial in which two therapies were tested in patients with long-standing anorexia nervosa [6] weight gain was modest but significant and there were significant improvements in depression and eating disorder symptoms. The two therapies were SSCM and cognitive behaviour therapy (CBT). SSCM is Specialist Supportive Clinical Management [25] and is a therapy that can be delivered by mental health staff without psychotherapy training. It mostly addresses eating disorder behaviours and has been used as a control therapy in several randomised trials [6, 26, 27] in which the results were surprisingly good, often doing as well as the more complex therapy being studied. Hence it has earned itself a place in the NICE guidelines [28]. Initially it was designed exclusively for anorexia nervosa and a variant (SSCM-ED) has been used in all eating disorders [29]. SSCM and SSCM-ED have no published manual but a manual for the latter can be obtained from the author of this chapter.

4.5 Physical risk monitoring

This is clearly required in anorexia nervosa of any duration, because without in patients can deteriorate and die from nutritional problems. For bulimia nervosa, the most common serious medical problems are electrolyte disturbances. Who should do the monitoring is a point of debate. When specialist eating disorder services are scarce and expensive, there is an argument for monitoring to be based in primary care. However, the staff in primary care require training in monitoring eating disorders and in what to do when a worrying finding, such as an abnormal ECG, is uncovered. Some general practitioners are reluctant to take on this work, and a possible model in the UK NHS might be to provide funding for primary care staff to provide this service, and a formal link with an eating disorders specialist to provide support and guidance when abnormalities are discovered. Unfortunately, this has not yet been achieved and care is thus often a source of tension between primary and specialist care. Methods for monitoring patients with eating disorders have been documented in MARSIPAN [30] and in Treasure [31]. For monitoring of physical problems which develop over time but do not usually threaten life, such as osteoporosis, the patient and doctor need to decide on whether and how often to monitor the conditions. Some have argued that as the sole effective treatment for osteoporosis due to anorexia nervosa is weight gain, and as we know it will get worse without increase in weight, repeated scans are not required. Others believe that knowing that the condition is deteriorating might provide an incentive to improve weight and secondly alerts patient, physician and family to the increasing possibility of fractures after trivial or no injury.

4.6 Family interventions

Many patients with SEED-AN and SEED-BN describe difficulties with their families as already described. The problems from the family members' point of view are how to respond to a serious eating disorder which does not seem to be getting better, without suffering from depression and other manifestations of stress, and without inadvertently making the eating disorder worse. For these families, collaborative caring [32] has a lot to offer, and has been shown [33] to result in lower distress levels in carers. Single or multiple family therapy might sometimes be indicated to help resolve some difficulties, although naturally the aim of therapy would be improving family functioning and quality of life, rather than curing the eating disorder, as it is in younger, short history patients [34].

4.7 Social and occupational interventions

As described above, social isolation is commonly described in patients with long term anorexia nervosa and bulimia nervosa. Patients are reluctant to eat with others and may turn down invitations to go out, preferring to stay at home and binge-eat. Attending a day service for treatment can be a first step in re-socialising and help to find appropriate voluntary work or educational courses can also be a useful aid to recreating a social network. Some patients, especially with anorexia nervosa, find that meeting other patients with the same condition can be more acceptable, because they do not need to explain their behaviour to others. However, while this may be helpful initially, it can result in further entrenchment of the eating disorder and if possible, wider social networks should be sought. The help of occupational therapy and nursing staff can be invaluable in this process. If a patient already has a career, or is mid way through a training, the staff can help them reintegrate and request observer status before going back to work or study. For certain occupations, such as dance or athletics, the patient needs to decide whether pursuing the former career is possible without the eating disorder becoming more severe.

5. Summary and conclusions

A substantial proportion of individuals with eating disorder fail to recover either because they have not had early access to treatment, or because they have not responded to such treatment. As time goes on the chances of recovery reduce but they never seem to reach zero, suggesting an asymptotic function underlying the chances of recovery with time. There is some evidence to suggest that over 3 years, anorexia nervosa, but not, apparently bulimia nervosa, may become more entrenched and resistant to treatment. Both conditions, however, profoundly affect quality of life and although the mortality is lower in bulimia nervosa, both conditions are associated with widespread disruption of physical health and psychological, family and social functioning. In long term eating disorders each of these realms require attention from professionals and from other informed individuals in families, who require adequate training and support, and the general public including ex-sufferers and charities such as BEAT. Severe and enduring eating disorders (SEED) should be recognised by the wider psychiatry community as deserving of attention and resources as much as other severe and enduring mental disorders so that the suffering endured by patients and their families as well as the costs incurred by individuals, families and society can be alleviated.

Acknowledgements

The author would like to thank Ms. Jessica Jackson, Ms. Maxine Hughes, and Ms. Giulia Guidetti for permission to quote qualitative interview subjects. The author also thanks Professor Elena Tomba and Ms. Valentina Gardini, University of Bologna, for permission to quote data in **Figure 2** and associated text.

Author details

Paul Robinson[1,2]

1 Orri, UK

2 University College London, UK

*Address all correspondence to: drpaulrobinson@gmail.com

References

[1] Department of Health and Social Care. A National Service Framework for Mental Health: Modern standards and service models. UK: Department of Health; 1999

[2] National Institute for Health and Care Excellence (NICE). Draft guideline scope: Rehabilitation in adults with severe and enduring mental illness. 2018. Available from: https://www.nice.org.uk/guidance/gid-ng10092/documents/draft-scope

[3] Ruggeri M, Leese M, Thornicroft G, Bisoffi G, Tansella M. Definition and prevalence of severe and persistent mental illness. The British Journal of Psychiatry. 2000;**177**(2):149-155

[4] Robinson P. Severe and Enduring Eating Disorder (SEED): Management of Complex Presentations of Anorexia and Bulimia Nervosa. Wiley: Chichester; 2009. p. 184

[5] American Psychiatric Association. Diagnostic and Statistical Manual of Mental Disorders. 5th ed. Washington, DC: American Psychiatric Association; 2013

[6] Touyz S, Le Grange D, Lacey H, Hay P, Smith R, Maguire S, et al. Treating severe and enduring anorexia nervosa: A randomized controlled trial. Psychological Medicine. 2013;**43**(12):2512

[7] Treasure J, Russell G. The case for early intervention in anorexia nervosa: Theoretical exploration of maintaining factors. The British Journal of Psychiatry. 2011;**199**(1):5-7

[8] Russell GF, Szmukler GI, Dare C, Eisler I. An evaluation of family therapy in anorexia nervosa and bulimia nervosa. Archives of General Psychiatry. 1987;**44**(12):1047-1056

[9] Theander S. Outcome and prognosis in anorexia nervosa and bulimia: Some results of previous investigations, compared with those of a Swedish long-term study. Journal of Psychiatric Research. 1985;**19**(2-3):493-508

[10] Deter HC, Herzog W. Anorexia nervosa in a long-term perspective: Results of the Heidelberg-Mannheim study. Psychosomatic Medicine. 1994;**56**(1):20-27

[11] Fichter MM, Quadflieg N, Hedlund S. Twelve-year course and outcome predictors of anorexia nervosa. The International Journal of Eating Disorders. 2006;**39**(2):87-100

[12] Herpertz-Dahlmann B, Muller B, Herpertz S, Heussen N. Prospective 10-year follow-up in adolescent anorexia nervosa—Course, outcome, psychiatric comorbidity, and psychosocial adaptation. Journal of Child Psychology and Psychiatry. 2001;**42**(5):603-612

[13] Ratnasuriya RH, Eisler I, Szmukler GI, Russell GF. Anorexia nervosa: Outcome and prognostic factors after 20 years. The British Journal of Psychiatry. 1991;**158**:495-502

[14] Strober M, Freeman R, Morrell W. The long-term course of severe anorexia nervosa in adolescents: Survival analysis of recovery, relapse, and outcome predictors over 10-15 years in a prospective study. The International Journal of Eating Disorders. 1997;**22**(4):339-360

[15] Wentz E, Gillberg C, Gillberg IC, Rastam M. Ten-year follow-up of adolescent-onset anorexia nervosa: Psychiatric disorders and overall functioning scales. Journal of Child Psychology and Psychiatry. 2001;**42**(5):613-622

[16] Wentz E, Gillberg IC, Anckarsater H, Gillberg C, Rastam M. Adolescent-onset anorexia nervosa: 18-year outcome.

The British Journal of Psychiatry. 2009;**194**(2):168-174

[17] Gardini V. When do Eating Disorders Become Severe and Enduring?. Unpublished Master degree dissertation, Supervisor Prof. Elena Tomba. Bologna: University of Bologna; 2019

[18] Robinson PH, Kukucska R, Guidetti G, Leavey G. Severe and enduring anorexia nervosa (SEED-AN): A qualitative study of patients with 20+ years of anorexia nervosa. European Eating Disorders Review. 2015;**23**(4):318-326

[19] Yager J. Management of patients with chronic, intractable eating disorders. In: Yager PS, editor. Clinical Manual of Eating Disorders. London: American Psychiatric Publishing; 2007

[20] Wonderlich S, Mitchell JE, Crosby RD, Myers TC, Kadlec K, Lahaise K, et al. Minimizing and treating chronicity in the eating disorders: A clinical overview. The International Journal of Eating Disorders. 2012;**45**(4):467-475

[21] Slade M. Mental illness and well-being: The central importance of positive psychology and recovery approaches. BMC Health Services Research. 2010;**10**:26

[22] Walsh BT, Wilson GT, Loeb KL, Devlin MJ, Pike KM, Roose SP, et al. Medication and psychotherapy in the treatment of bulimia nervosa. The American Journal of Psychiatry. 1997;**154**(4):523-531

[23] Norris ML, Spettigue W, Buchholz A, Henderson KA, Gomez R, Maras D, et al. Olanzapine use for the adjunctive treatment of adolescents with anorexia nervosa. Journal of Child and Adolescent Psychopharmacology. 2011;**21**(3):213-220

[24] Fairburn CG, Cooper Z, Doll HA, O'Connor ME, Bohn K, Hawker DM, et al. Transdiagnostic cognitive-behavioral therapy for patients with eating disorders: A two-site trial with 60-week follow-up. The American Journal of Psychiatry. 2009;**166**(3):311-319

[25] McIntosh VV, Jordan J, Luty SE, Carter FA, McKenzie JM, Bulik CM, et al. Specialist supportive clinical management for anorexia nervosa. The International Journal of Eating Disorders. 2006;**39**(8):625-632

[26] Schmidt U, Renwick B, Lose A, Kenyon M, Dejong H, Broadbent H, et al. The MOSAIC study: Comparison of the Maudsley model of treatment for adults with anorexia nervosa (MANTRA) with Specialist Supportive Clinical Management (SSCM) in outpatients with anorexia nervosa or eating disorder not otherwise specified, anorexia nervosa type: Study protocol for a randomized controlled trial. Trials. 2013;**14**:160

[27] McIntosh VV, Jordan J, Carter JD, Frampton CM, McKenzie JM, Latner JD, et al. Psychotherapy for transdiagnostic binge eating: A randomized controlled trial of cognitive-behavioural therapy, appetite-focused cognitive-behavioural therapy, and schema therapy. Psychiatry Research. 2016;**240**:412-420

[28] National Institute for Health and Care Excellence. Eating disorders: Recognition and treatment. NG69; 2017

[29] Robinson P, Hellier J, Barrett B, Barzdaitiene D, Bateman A, Bogaardt A, et al. The NOURISHED randomised controlled trial comparing mentalisation-based treatment for eating disorders (MBT-ED) with specialist supportive clinical management (SSCM-ED) for patients with eating disorders and symptoms of borderline personality disorder. Trials. 2016;**17**(1):549

[30] Royal College of Psychiatrists. MARSIPAN CR189. London; 2014

[31] Treasure J. A Guide to the Medical Risk Assessment for Eating Disorders. 2009; Available from: https://www.kcl.ac.uk/ioppn/depts/pm/research/eatingdisorders/resources/GUIDETOMEDICALRISKASSESSMENT.pdf [Accessed: March 31, 2019]

[32] Treasure J, Sepulveda AR, Whitaker W, Todd G, Lopez C, Whitney J. Collaborative care between professionals and non-professionals in the management of eating disorders: A description of workshops focussed on interpersonal maintaining factors. European Eating Disorders Review. 2007;**15**(1):24-34

[33] Whitney J, Murphy T, Landau S, Gavan K, Todd G, Whitaker W, et al. A practical comparison of two types of family intervention: An exploratory RCT of family day workshops and individual family work as a supplement to inpatient care for adults with anorexia nervosa. European Eating Disorders Review. 2012;**20**(2):142-150

[34] Blessitt E, Voulgari S, Eisler I. Family therapy for adolescent anorexia nervosa. Current Opinion in Psychiatry. 2015;**28**(6):455-460